Plant Based Body Transformation

A Comprehensive Beginners Guide to Building Muscle & Shredding Fat

Lisa Aguilar

© Copyright 2023 - All rights reserved.

The content contained within this book may not be reproduced, duplicated or transmitted without direct written permission from the author or the publisher.

Under no circumstances will any blame or legal responsibility be held against the publisher, or author, for any damages, reparation, or monetary loss due to the information contained within this book, either directly or indirectly.

Legal Notice:

This book is copyright protected. It is only for personal use. You cannot amend, distribute, sell, use, quote or paraphrase any part, or the content within this book, without the consent of the author or publisher.

Disclaimer Notice:

Please note the information contained within this document is for educational and entertainment purposes only. All effort has been executed to present accurate, up to date, reliable, complete information. No warranties of any kind are declared or implied. Readers acknowledge that the author is not engaged in the rendering of legal, financial, medical or professional advice. The content within this book has been derived from various sources. Please consult a licensed professional before attempting any techniques outlined in this book.

By reading this document, the reader agrees that under no circumstances is the author responsible for any losses, direct or indirect, that are incurred as a result of the use of the information contained within this document, including, but not limited to, errors, omissions, or inaccuracies.

Table of Contents

INTRODUCTION 1

CHAPTER 1: UNDERSTANDING THE PLANT-BASED ADVANTAGE 5

    THE NUTRITIONAL RICHNESS OF PLANT-BASED FOODS 6
        Plant Protein and Its Muscle-Building Potential 9
        Harnessing the Power of Phytonutrients 12

CHAPTER 2: SETTING THE FOUNDATION—GOAL SETTING AND PLANNING 15

    DEFINING YOUR FITNESS OBJECTIVES 16
        Creating a Personalized Nutrition and Training Plan 19
        Tracking Progress Effectively 23

CHAPTER 3: CRAFTING A PLANT-POWERED PLATE 27

    THE CORE COMPONENTS OF A BALANCED PLANT-BASED MEAL 28
        Meeting Macronutrient and Micronutrient Needs 30
        Calculating Your Macros and Designing Meals for Muscle Growth and Fat Loss 32

CHAPTER 4: PLANT PROTEIN MASTERY 35

    EXPLORING DIVERSE PLANT-BASED PROTEIN SOURCES 36
        Proper Timing and Quantity of Protein Intake 40
        Combining Proteins for Different Amino Acid Options 41

CHAPTER 5: FUELING YOUR WORKOUTS: PRE-, INTRA-, AND POSTNUTRITION 43

    ENERGIZING YOUR SESSIONS WITH SMART, PREWORKOUT MEALS 43
        Navigating Intraworkout Nutrition 46
        Optimizing Recovery with Postworkout Meals 48

CHAPTER 6: THE ROLE OF CARBOHYDRATES IN MUSCLE BUILDING AND FAT LOSS 51

    CARBOHYDRATES AS PERFORMANCE FUEL 52
        Tailoring Carb Intake to Your Fitness Goals 55
        Balancing Carbs to Prevent Fat Gain 56

CHAPTER 7: EMBRACING HEALTHY FATS 59

The Importance of Essential Fatty Acids 60
Incorporating Nutrient-Dense Fats Into Your Diet 61
Embracing Hormonal Balance and Recovery 63

CHAPTER 8: STRATEGIC SUPPLEMENTATION FOR VEGANS 65

Identifying Potential Nutritional Gaps 66
Vegan-Friendly Supplements for Muscle Building and Fat Loss 71
Maximizing Absorption and Effectiveness 74

CHAPTER 9: EFFECTIVE TRAINING STRATEGIES 77

Designing Resistance Training Programs for Muscle Gain 77
Incorporating Cardiovascular Training for Weight Loss 81

CHAPTER 10: RECOVERING AS A PLANT-BASED ATHLETE 85

Prioritizing Sleep and Health 86
Managing Stress and Cortisol Levels 87
Plant-Based Recovery Techniques and Strategies 90

CHAPTER 11: TROUBLESHOOTING AND OVERCOMING PLATEAUS 93

Identifying Common Challenges in a Vegan Diet 93
Adjusting Nutrition and Training for Continued Progress 95
Mental Strategies to Stay Motivated 96

CONCLUSION 99

BONUS CHAPTER: RECIPES 101

GLOSSARY 109

REFERENCES 111

Introduction

We live in an age of misinformation, where we are surrounded by myths that we easily take as facts. One of those myths is that vegetarianism and veganism aren't good for fitness. "You need protein if you want to build muscle," a lot of people walk around saying, "so you can't build muscle by eating a plant-based diet." This, however, is patently untrue. Not only is a plant-based diet great for building muscle and losing fat, but it's also better for your workouts. In fact, there are a lot of health and fitness benefits that come with eating a plant-based diet that many people either overlook or simply don't know about. There are a lot more people, though, who are all too aware of these benefits. That's why more and more athletes, including professional athletes, have been going vegetarian or even vegan in recent years. A recent study, for example, found that 34.7% of all long-distance runners are vegetarian, whereas 20.9% of them are vegan. That means less than half—specifically 44.4%—of all long-distance runners are omnivores (Wirnitzer et al., 2022).

Long-distance runners aren't the only athletes who seem to have taken a liking to vegetarianism and veganism. Many others have as well, from climbers such as James Parsley to weight lifters like Patrik Baboumian, Jehina Malik, and more. This is because more and more athletes are coming to recognize that not only are plant-based diets good for them, but they also improve their performance significantly. This is actually something that has been known to scientists since the 1890s (Greger, 2023). A study was conducted back then among weight lifters, examining how their eating habits impacted their ability to lift. The results were shocking to a lot of people because the study found that plant-based athletes were able to lift 80% more weight than athletes who were omnivores. The implications of this study were reconfirmed in a famous study that was conducted by Yale University a century later. This study found that vegetarian athletes' endurance levels were far greater than those who were omnivores (Lynch et al., 2016).

Whatever endurance tests were flung at them, plant-based athletes generally did at least five times as well as their meat-eating contemporaries.

Eating a plant-based diet, which includes consuming things like legumes and whole grains, is great for improving an athlete's performance. It comes with many other benefits too. For instance, plant-based foods are very nutrient rich. Not only are all those vegetables and fruits you eat packed with vitamins and minerals, but they also have lots of antioxidants in them. Antioxidants are known for helping to remove toxins from your body—hence the name. They're also known for helping with athletic recovery. Eating a vegetable- and fruit-heavy diet can reduce muscle soreness, make your muscles recover more quickly post-workout by reducing inflammation, and speed up muscle regeneration (Adidas Runtastic Team, 2022). So, athletes who prioritize plant-based foods tend to recover more quickly after their training sessions and games, as well as play stronger and run faster in general.

A plant-based diet also improves athletes' hydration levels. All human beings need to stay hydrated to survive (Sautter, 2023). That means drinking a certain amount of water per day. Athletes, however, need a little more water than regular human beings since they sweat out what they drink on a pretty regular basis. Drinking water, though, isn't the only way to hydrate yourself. Eating more fruits and vegetables can significantly help with this, seeing as they contain a lot of water in and of themselves. As a rule, plant-based foods are water rich, as well as low in fat and calories. So, not only do they keep you hydrated, but they make it easier for you to manage your weight or even lose weight if that's what you're trying to do.

Plant-based foods aren't just water rich. They're rich in fiber, too. Fiber is a type of carbohydrate (carb) that cannot be broken down by the enzymes in your digestive system. As such, it usually just passes through your digestive system and is expelled from your body, taking any harmful toxins that may have entered your system along with it. If you want to have a good digestive system, then you need to eat plenty of fiber-rich foods. In other words, you have to eat lots of plant-based foods. This way, you can increase your nutrition intake, keep your gut healthy, and rid your body of any and all harmful toxins.

A final advantage of a plant-based diet might be that it actually reduces your risk of developing some sort of chronic disease, like type 2 diabetes and various heart diseases. In recent years, it's even been discovered that a plant-based diet can help prevent certain types of cancer, thanks to all the nutrients and fiber that can be found in such foods (Burke et al., 2015).

With all this being the case, is it really all that surprising that more and more athletes—and nonathletes, for that matter—have been turning toward a plant-based diet? Not really. Looking at the matter objectively, it's easy to see that a plant-based diet can be very good for both your health and your performance levels. A number of people might object to this observation. They might be under the impression that a plant-based diet can't be good for you because it denies you one essential nutrient: protein. This, however, is yet another myth about a plant-based diet and one that can be easily disproven at that. You see, the recommended daily level of protein for a regular human being is 0.8 grams per kilogram of body weight. You don't have to eat two steaks per day to meet this requirement. In fact, you'd be going well over your daily protein requirement levels if you were to do that. All you have to do is eat some lentils, seeds, nuts, whole grains, or beans every day, and you'll be good to go.

Another interesting myth about plant-based diets is that they're too restrictive. A plant-based diet, though, is only as restrictive or expansive as you make it. Say that you're going to prepare some broccoli. If the only way you know to prepare broccoli is to steam it, then you are undeniably restricting your diet. If you're willing to try other recipes, on the other hand, and throw in different ingredients and spices, then you'll suddenly find that you have a lot more recipes to work with than you thought. This is especially true when you factor in all the different food substitutes, like dates for sugar, cheese made out of nuts, or even tofu. Truthfully, there's only one thing that can limit you in the kitchen once you've opted for a plant-based diet, and that's your own imagination. It's as simple as that.

Plainly put, a plant-based diet can be incredibly delicious, versatile, and very healthy for you as both a person and an athlete. This, of course, only holds true if you know the right way to go about crafting your very own plant-based diet. What makes for a good, healthy plant-based diet then? How can you ensure you maintain a balanced diet while opting for plant-based foods? How can you make sure that you're choosing foods that will enhance and improve your performance levels while looking out for your health? More importantly, how can you craft the perfect plant-based diet for you, thus meeting your own specific needs and sparking the kind of transformation you are looking for? Let's find out!

Chapter 1:

Understanding the Plant-Based Advantage

Einstein once said, "If the whole world adopts vegetarianism, it can change the destiny of humankind." Einstein was one of the smartest people to ever walk the Earth, as you know. He was also a vegetarian (Richards, 2023). Einstein decided to become a vegetarian late in life. As a man of science, his decision wasn't based on trends or fashions. Rather, it was based on the objective fact that vegetarianism was simply better for human health, as well as for the world itself.

Not everyone in the world agrees with Albert Einstein, of course, but a great many people do. What's more, the number of people who convert to vegetarianism and even veganism seems to increase year by year. Today, 1.5 billion people maintain a vegetarian, that is to say, plant-based diet. That means that 22% of the world's population refuses to eat meat, and that figure seems only to be growing, if the current size of the plant-based market is anything to go by. Currently, the plant-based market is worth $1.4 billion globally, which is 74% larger than what it used to be three years ago (Van Niekerk, 2023).

Why is this the case? Why are more and more people turning away from meat and opting for plant-based options and lifestyles? Why is a plant-based diet better for you, and why, for that matter, is it better for humankind, as Einstein said?

The Nutritional Richness of Plant-Based Foods

Truthfully, there are a great many reasons for this. Some of them have to do with the way in which plant-based foods impact your health. Others have to do with the environmental impact that moving away from a meat-based diet brings with it. You see, plant-based foods are incredibly rich in nutrients, including antioxidants, vitamins, and minerals. Your body needs all these nutrients to be able to perform at an optimal level. Those nutrients, in turn, affect your body in a variety of ways. For example, eating a plant-based diet is known to reduce blood pressure. The nutrients found in such foods keep your blood pressure and cholesterol levels from rising the way they do when you eat meat-based diets. At least, that's what studies indicate (Yokoyama et al., 2014). One study, for example, has shown that vegetarians are 34% less at risk of developing hypertension than nonvegetarians (Chuang et al., 2016).

The nutrients that are found in plant-based foods don't just lower your blood pressure and cholesterol levels; they also lower inflammation. Inflammation is a kind of healing process in your body. When a foreign object, such as a splinter or a microorganism like a virus, gets in your body, white blood cells are immediately sent out to deal with it. These white blood cells fight against the foreign invaders they encounter. As they do, the tissue upon which they're waging that battle, like your throat, becomes red and swollen.

That sore throat right there is inflammation. Certain things, like added sugars and unhealthy fats like the kind found in hot dogs, can worsen inflammation. Others, like vitamin D, can soothe it. As you might have guessed by now, most of those nutrients can be found in plant-based foods. Since plant-based foods reduce inflammation, it shouldn't be all that surprising to find out that they help reduce arthritis pain. Arthritis pain is typically related to inflammation in the joints, so the lower the level of inflammation, the better you'll feel, and the more easily you'll be able to move around (Clinton et al., 2015).

The nutrients in plant-based foods can do all sorts of additional things, like improve kidney function and lower your risk of developing diabetes. They can, therefore, not only prevent chronic kidney disease but also reduce mortality rates among individuals with this disease. Eating a nutrient-rich plant-based diet can even reverse type 2 diabetes over time. Meanwhile, eating red meat can increase your risk of developing diabetes by as much as 23% (Talaei et al., 2017).

Then there's the way plant-based foods impact heart disease. Plant-based foods are rich in fiber, which is necessary for the functioning of your digestive system. At the same time, they're low in saturated fats—the kind of fat you typically want to avoid, as you'll see later—and have no dietary cholesterol to speak of. Hence, they're extremely good for your heart health. They can help you keep your cholesterol levels low, making it hard for you to develop heart disease.

A plant-based diet is also very good for your brain health in that it wards your brain against dementia and other kinds of cognitive impairment. This is all thanks to the folates, vitamins, and antioxidants that are found in plant-based foods, which are known to have cognitive benefits like improving your long- and short-term memory and expanding your attention span (Jiang et al., 2017).

Plant-based diets can be beneficial for individuals with thyroid conditions such as Hashimoto's thyroiditis and hypothyroidism due to several reasons. These diets are typically rich in antioxidants, vitamins, minerals, and dietary fiber, which can help reduce inflammation and support overall thyroid health. A study published in the journal *Frontiers in Endocrinology* in 2019 noted that a plant-based diet can have anti-inflammatory effects and potentially lower autoimmune responses associated with Hashimoto's thyroiditis. Furthermore, plant-based diets are often lower in saturated fats and cholesterol, which can help manage weight and improve heart health, both important factors for individuals with thyroid conditions. The ample supply of nutrients from plant foods can also promote better digestion and absorption of essential nutrients, ultimately supporting thyroid function. While plant-based diets can be a valuable addition to a comprehensive thyroid management plan, it's essential for individuals with these conditions to work closely with healthcare professionals to tailor their dietary choices to their specific needs and monitor their thyroid function regularly.

Travel a little farther down south, and you'll find that a plant-based diet is good for your gut health, too. Your guts are filled with all sorts of good bacteria. These bacteria help you to ferment and digest your food, so you want to have a lot of them in there. These bacteria also feed on specific kinds of nutrients. Without those nutrients, they starve and start dying off. The kinds of nutrients your good bacteria snack on can mostly be found in plant-based foods. By prioritizing this kind of food, then, you can support the good bacteria colonies that can be found in your gut. Thus, you can not only improve your digestion but also strengthen your immune system and hormonal balance since studies show that your gut microbiome—the bacteria populations in your gut—drastically affects both (Wu & Wu, 2012).

The link between eating and weight management being what it is, you won't be too shocked to hear that a plant-based diet can make weight loss and management a whole lot easier for you. There's ample evidence to prove as much. According to one such study, the average non-vegetarian male's body mass index (BMI) averages around 28.8, which is the BMI of someone who is overweight. The average vegan's BMI, on the other hand, ranges around 23.6, which means that they're typically not overweight. As a rule, then, individuals on plant-based diets weigh less. They also lose weight more easily. Overweight individuals over the age of 65, for instance, lose around 9.5 pounds per year when they switch to plant-based diets (National Heart, Lung, and Blood Institute, 2019). Of course, all of this is contingent on eating healthy plant-based foods. If you're eating deep-fried eggplant and french fries every day, the odds are that none of this is going to apply to you.

That a plant-based diet makes weight management easier might not have been surprising but finding out that this type of diet can actually reduce your risk of developing certain types of cancer probably will be. More specifically, a plant-based diet can protect you against one-third of all cancer types out there, including gastrointestinal, breast, prostate, and colorectal cancers. Considering most of these cancer types have to do with your digestive system, this effect can very easily be attributed to the many nutrients to be found in plant-based foods, can it not?

It should be obvious by now that eating a plant-based diet is much better for your health and well-being than a meat-based one. That a plant-based diet can actually expand your lifespan, though, may not be as evident. Luckily, studies can prove even that. Recent research indicates that plant-based diets lower human mortality by as much as 25% (Kim et al., 2019).

Plant Protein and Its Muscle-Building Potential

Switching to a plant-based diet can have a great many benefits to offer you, especially if you're an athlete. There are some athletes who might be hesitant to do so because they're under the impression that plant-based foods will stymie their efforts to build muscle. This, however, isn't even close to the truth. Maintaining a plant-based diet wouldn't impede your efforts to bulk up and get stronger. If anything, it would support them.

When you're working out, you create microscopic tears all over your muscles. These tears then need to be healed, and your body gets to work doing that. As it knits your muscles back together, it makes sure to add some extra layers of muscle over those tears. In this way, your body tries to make your muscles more resilient to future tears, and in doing so, it causes you to bulk up and get stronger. Your body essentially needs amino acids, the building blocks that are found in proteins, to be able to create muscle fibers in this way and repair microtears.

This is why eating protein is so important, but does that protein really have to come from meat? Not really. Studies show that those who stick to plant-based diets are able to build muscles the exact same way that those who stick to omnivorous diets can. This is clear evidence that meat isn't necessary to build muscle. All you really need is protein, and you can make sure you can get enough of that by eating a diverse variety of plant-based foods. The key word there is "diverse." Do you remember how proteins are made of amino acids? Well, there are 20 different kinds of amino acids out there, and your body needs pretty much all of them, especially when repairing microtears. The problem ⸴ that different kinds of them exist in different kinds of plant-b foods. So, if you only eat lentils, for example, you'll only be eight different kinds of amino acids and deprive yourself of ⸴

make sure you're meeting all your amino acid needs, you have to eat colorful, varied meals made up of many different plant proteins.

You have a wide array of options to choose from when it comes to plant protein, such as

- seeds and kernels
- nuts
- peanut butter
- spirulina
- legumes and beans
- tempeh
- tofu
- fresh green vegetables like artichokes
- protein powder (de Groot, 2020)

These kinds of plant-based foods tend to be high in protein, though fresh green vegetables contain the least amount. Hence, you can meet all your amino acid needs by adding these to your diet. Making a green smoothie with some protein powder in it for the morning, having an apple with peanut butter on it as an afternoon snack, eating a three-bean salad for lunch, and having a tofu burger at night is just one example of how you might incorporate different plant-based proteins into your daily diet.

Having said all that, there are a couple of rules you need to follow when switching to a plant-based diet. These easy-to-follow rules can ensure that you meet your protein requirements properly and don't deprive your body of anything it needs. Your first rule is to check how much protein and other nutrients specific ingredients contain as you're planning your meals. As a most basic example, brown rice only contains 5 grams of protein per every 0.17 ounces. So, relying on it exclusively for your protein needs isn't a good idea, that is unless you mean to eat bowl upon bowl of brown rice. This is especially true when you consider that an average 150-pound individual would need between 81 and 136 grams of protein per day to be able to build muscle (Satrazemis, 2022).

Since you need to eat a specific amount of protein to be able to build muscle, that means you also need to track your daily protein intake (*Can You Build Muscle with Plant-Based Protein?*, n.d.). That is rule number two. The good news is tracking your protein intake is pretty easy to do, especially these days. There are many free apps you can use for just this purpose. Of course, keeping track of your protein intake doesn't mean writing down "a handful of brown rice" in your app, the same way your grandmother would write "a dash of paprika" in her recipe book, expecting everyone to understand the exact amount she means. Rather, it means properly measuring your ingredients while they're still raw. This will yield the most accurate information as to how much food and protein you're consuming.

Muscle building while eating a plant-based diet requires one other thing: consistency. This applies to both your nutrition and your workout habits. If you're not regularly doing strength training, then you're probably not going to be able to build muscle no matter how much protein you consume. Likewise, if you're not eating a sufficient amount of protein on a regular basis, then you won't be able to develop any muscle mass, seeing as your body will be deprived of the amino acids it needs to do so.

Consistency, then, is key here, as is making sure to lift heavy. As you build muscle, you will obviously get stronger. After a certain point, the weights that used to give you trouble will start feeling almost feather-light to you. That means they'll no longer be enough to create microtears. Hence, they won't be enough to make your body create more muscle fibers. You can circumnavigate this issue by gradually increasing the weights you're working out with. Alternatively, you can increase the number of sets and reps once your body has gotten used to the weights you're working out with. This can push your muscles beyond their limit and create new microtears, thus helping you to grow stronger. These are two ways to progressively overload your muscles to continue to make progress toward your goal.

Last but not least, if you want to build muscle, then you're going to have to not only hit your daily protein goal but your daily calorie goal as well. As a rule, plant-based foods tend to have fewer calories than other types of foods. Given that, you have to eat a lot more of them in order to be able to meet your goals. Otherwise, you will hit a calorie deficit, which not only won't help you gain muscle but it'll cause you to lose weight as well, no matter how hard you work out. Someone on a plant-based diet who wants to build muscle typically needs to consume about 2,500 calories per day (Cheeke, 2021). All those calories, however, should come from plant-based foods and not, say, two giant pizzas. This is because plant-based foods will contain nutrients that will aid with muscle regeneration and soreness, whereas other types of food usually won't.

Harnessing the Power of Phytonutrients

Speaking of nutrients that support muscle building, there's a kind that's especially good at this: phytonutrients. Phytonutrients are a kind of chemical that plants exclusively produce that is really beneficial for you. Otherwise known as antioxidants, phytonutrients fight off something called "free radicals." Free radicals is the catch-all term for harmful chemical substances that get into your body and weaken your immune system or interfere with the general functioning of your body. Luckily, what you need to do to get rid of these substances is pretty obvious: Eat lots of plant-based foods with lots of antioxidants in them.

Just as there are different types of amino acids out there, there are different types of phytonutrients you need to consume as well. Chief among these are magnesium, selenium, zinc, copper, vitamin C, vitamin E, and beta-carotene, which is a substance that's pretty closely related to vitamin A. These minerals and vitamins all fall under the phytonutrients umbrella, and they're not just good at fighting free radicals. They're also really good at improving your postworkout recovery and enhancing your ability to build your muscles. This is because antioxidants bind and deactivate any free radicals that are generated in your body following a workout session. In doing so, they prevent them from damaging your muscle cells. Second, they actually strengthen the cell membranes—that is to say, protective walls—of your muscle cells, thereby making them more resilient against free radicals. These effects not only enable your body to create more muscle fibers faster, but they also lessen things like muscle soreness. In other words, they help you to recover quicker from your workouts and hit the gym again without much trouble.

So, which plant-based foods are high in phytonutrients? Put another way, which foods do you need to eat to make sure you have plenty of antioxidants in your system? The answer to that question depends on what kind of phytonutrient you're dealing with. If you want to eat more magnesium, for example, then you'll have to add legumes, whole grains, and leafy greens to the menu. If, on the other hand, you want more selenium, you'll have to eat more whole grains and seafood. For copper, you'll need to prioritize nuts, legumes, and whole grains. Meanwhile, introducing more vitamin E to your diet means eating plenty of nuts and seeds, as well as using vegetable oils in your cooking. For vitamin C, you'll obviously turn to citrus fruits such as oranges or make juices out of them. You can also find plenty of vitamin C in tomatoes, peppers, cabbage, berries, and cantaloupe. As for beta-carotene, this is found in plenty of plant-based foods, including

- kale
- collard
- turnips
- beets
- tomatoes
- spinach
- broccoli
- carrots
- sweet potatoes

- peppers
- papaya
- apricots
- mangos
- cantaloupes

As important as eating these different plant-based foods is for your health, they won't do much to help your efforts to build muscle if you're not working out regularly. Nutrition and your workout sessions need to go hand in hand. That is the only way you'll ever be able to get any results. Having said that, you can't just go with any old workout because working out isn't a one-size-fits-all practice. Rather, it's something that should be tailor-made for the individual because every human being's needs are different. No one's metabolism, for instance, works at quite the same speed as another's. So, how do you go about crafting the perfect muscle-building workout routine for yourself? Let's find out.

Chapter 2:

Setting the Foundation—Goal Setting and Planning

Working out regularly and getting into shape is something that everyone should do, no matter what their age, if they want to be as healthy as they can be. Getting fit, though, can be a little challenging, at least if you don't put a good plan in place and set some sound fitness goals for yourself. This is because a good fitness plan can serve as your roadmap. It can save you a great deal of time when you're at the gym, thinking *What should I do next?* It can keep you from engaging in unnecessary sets and reps, working muscles that you've already worked. In other words, it can make it so that you can walk into a workout session knowing full well what you're going to do and how you're going to do it.

Meanwhile, setting fitness goals for yourself can provide you with important milestones to work toward. By sticking to your workout plan, you'll be able to meet those milestones one by one. Each milestone you meet will encourage and motivate you to keep going. At the same time, they'll give you the ability to track your progress. Naturally, all this is dependent on your ability to create the right plan for yourself, as well as set the right goals for you? What does that mean, though? How can you tell whether your fitness plan is a good one or not or whether your goals are right for you, for that matter?

Defining Your Fitness Objectives

Your fitness objectives are primarily the progress and performance goals that you set for yourself. They're benchmarks to meet in your fitness journey, as well as measures you can use to see how far you've come in both the short and long terms. Your goals, however, have to be worded and structured in a specific way for this to truly be the case. Otherwise, they'll be too vague for you to be able to meet. This is why a lot of athletes like setting SMART fitness goals for themselves. SMART goals are goals that are

- **S**pecific

- **M**easurable

- **A**chievable

- **R**elevant

- **T**ime-bound (*Physical Activity–Setting Yourself Goals*, 2012)

It's important that your fitness goals meet these SMART criteria because otherwise, you likely won't ever be able to meet them. To start with the first of these characteristics, your fitness goals need to be specific because such objectives give you a very firm idea of what you need to achieve. This, in turn, helps you to quickly and clearly see what you need to do to meet that goal. "Get fit" may sound like a good goal, but it's a very vague one when you think about it. I mean, what does "fit" mean in this case? How will you know when you've become "fit"? What is your vision of "fit?" How will you know when you've met your goal?

Odds are, your answers to those questions are "I don't know" or "I'm not sure," which is why you need your goals to be specific. You can make sure that that's the case by setting goals that answer five specific questions:

- What will you be doing?
- How will you be doing it?
- Where will you be doing it?
- When will you be doing it by?
- Who will you be doing it with?

As an example, "Swim 10 laps by yourself at the local swimming pool twice a week, every week, without stopping" is a specific goal that answers all five of these questions. Hence, it leaves no room for doubt as to what your goal is and how you can achieve it.

Then there's measurability. Your fitness goals need to be as measurable as humanly possible for two reasons. The first is that measurable goals enable you to track your progress. The second is that such goals are immensely motivating because they show you how much progress you've made over time. This can drive you to keep going forward, even when the going gets tough, and even if you don't particularly enjoy working out.

As for achievability, that refers to how realistic the goals you set for yourself are. If you haven't been working out for the past 20 years and have only just started going to the gym, then odds are, you're not going to be able to do 50 push-ups in one go. If that's the immediate goal you set for yourself, you, therefore, won't be able to meet it, and you'll get disheartened as a result. You might even quit working out altogether. What if your initial goal was to be able to do 10 push-ups in a row? You'd be able to meet this goal a lot more easily, right? After you have, you could set your next goal of doing 15 push-ups in a row, then 20, and then 30. You can keep going like that, gradually increasing the number of push-ups you do with each training session.

Your fitness goals also need to be relevant, which means that they need to fit in with your lifestyle choices, health conditions, and the like. If you're working late into the night every weekday, for example, and get home late, then aiming to work out for an hour every night probably won't be very doable. This is especially true if you find that you come home drained and too exhausted to move at the end of the day. Scheduling a 20-minute walk for yourself during your one-hour-long lunch break or waking up an hour earlier each day to complete your cardio or weightlifting, on the other hand, will be far more doable for you.

Last but not least, any fitness goal you set for yourself should be time-bound. That means that they should indicate precisely when you mean to achieve that goal. That way, you can steadily track your progress and keep your motivation levels up. Even meeting small milestones can be vital for this. You'll also be able to stick more closely to your training plan since the time frame you give yourself will keep you from slacking off.

Setting SMART goals for yourself can be immensely effective. The key to them, though, is to set new goals for yourself once you've met your old ones. That is to only way to keep moving forward. Likewise, it's important that you regularly assess your goals to make sure they're realistic and achievable for you at that given time. If you find that you're particularly struggling with a goal, then perhaps you might consider adjusting it or dividing it into smaller goals.

Making your goals measurable is a great practice because it makes it easier for you to reassess them periodically. It gives you the ability to ask questions like, "Have I been able to meet this goal yet?" or "How quickly have I been able to achieve a milestone?" The honest answers you give to such questions allow you to make changes as necessary. For instance, if you find that you're meeting a goal too quickly, you can make it a little more challenging for yourself. If, on the other hand, it's too hard, then you can change it accordingly.

This kind of flexibility is vital when you're setting fitness goals for yourself and trying to meet them. Obviously, this is something that'll affect the fitness plan you craft for yourself, too. Hence, it's important that you create the kind of fitness plan that can be changed as necessary. At the end of the day, a rigid training plan will be one that you won't be able to abide by, no matter how hard you try. Adaptability isn't the only rule of law where training and nutrition plans are concerned, though. A myriad of other factors goes into this matter as well, as you'll soon see.

Creating a Personalized Nutrition and Training Plan

Your first step to creating fitness and nutrition plans that work for you is to consider your fitness goals carefully. That way, your plans will lead to your goals directly. To start with your fitness or training plan, your first step is to assess your current fitness level. This includes taking a look at your conditioning, muscle strength, flexibility, and overall body composition (*5 Steps to Start a Fitness Program*, 2019). You can assess these things by

- taking a look at how quick your pulse is after you've been walking for a mile

- how long it takes you to walk a mile

- how many push-ups you can do in one go

- how far you can reach when sitting on the floor with your legs extended before you

- what your waist circumference is when you measure it just above your hipbones

- what your body mass index (BMI) is

Once you've evaluated your fitness level, you can take another look at your goals, especially your main goal. Why are you working out in the first place? Is it to lose weight or maintain your current weight? Is it for your heart health, or is it that you want to become stronger? Are you training for something specific, like a marathon? Gaining clarity on your overarching goal will not only prove motivating, but it'll also help you get a lot more specific in your training plan.

As for the training plan itself, experts generally agree that a normal individual should get 150 minutes of moderate-level aerobic—meaning cardio—activity per week. Alternatively, you can get just 75 minutes of vigorous aerobic activity per week. This is just for maintaining your health and current weight, though. If you want to lose weight, then you'll have to work out 300 minutes per week at a moderate level instead (*5 Steps to Start a Fitness Program*, 2019). The difference here has to do with how fast your workout routine gets your heart pumping. Moderate activity should elevate your pulse and quicken your breathing enough that you can still say a few words while you talk but shouldn't be able to hold long conversations. Vigorous activity should get your heart beating really quickly, make you sweat a lot, and make you start breathing quickly enough that you can't speak. As a rule, you should do 75 minutes of this vigorous cardio per week, though how you divide that up among your days is up to you.

All that being said, your fitness plan shouldn't get your heart pounding immediately. Rather, your daily workout routine should focus on gradually raising your heartbeat and breathing rates. That means that you should start slow and increase your workout difficulty as time goes on. If you've ever been to the gym or done home workouts, as many of us have done during the pandemic, you know that you execute certain workout moves. You do specific moves in groups of three or four. These groups are called sets. Three or four sets typically follow after one another before you pause momentarily and repeat your sets. Another word for this is doing "reps." Your workout routine for the day should be made up of different kinds of sets. Your aim should be to include a warm-up set followed by three to four working sets, with your last set continuing to failure—failure on your form, failure on the positive movement, or failure on the negative movement. The workout routine you craft for yourself, then, should be made up of a variety of movements. This will ensure you work different muscle groups throughout your body and keep things from getting too boring for you.

Variety isn't just something that applies to your daily routine but to your weekly fitness plan, too. Your fitness plan, you see, should be made up of different activities like swimming, jogging, CrossFit, going to the gym, and more. This way, you can do cardio exercises and strength—that is to say, muscle training—exercises regularly. A healthy body requires both types of activity. So, doing just one or the other isn't a very good idea. The key thing to remember when deciding on your activities is to choose ones that work for your lifestyle and that you actually enjoy. If you make swimming a part of your fitness plan, but the nearest swimming pool is a two-hour drive from where you live and work, then that's not going to be very doable for you. Likewise, if you dislike swimming or find it boring, then you probably won't stick with it in the long run. By choosing activities that you enjoy, you can decrease the likelihood that you'll quit working out halfway through the year. Thus, you'll be able to keep your fitness plan realistic and turn it into a lifelong habit.

A lot of people are under the impression that having a fitness plan means you have to take care of all your daily exercise in one go. Given that, they become liable to skip exercising on particularly busy days, saying, "I don't have time to work out for a full hour today." This excuse would have been understandable if you really weren't allowed to break up your exercise routine into, say, 10-30-minute chunks. That, however, is not the case. You can break up your exercise into such chunks and take care of them whenever you have a moment throughout the day. You can squeeze in some stretching and strength exercises after you wake up, for instance, pencil in a 30-minute walk in the afternoon and then work out an additional 30 minutes before you go to bed at night. The following day, when your schedule is freer, you can work out continuously for 45 minutes or an hour.

What if you don't have the stamina to work out for that long yet? That's perfectly alright. In that case, you can keep your initial workout sessions shorter. You can slowly keep adding more activities to your fitness plan, thereby extending your workout time as your stamina keeps increasing. You can also up the difficulty level of your moves or the number of reps you do as time goes by. That being said, you should immediately stop working out if you feel any pain that's not the regular kind of muscle burn that comes with exercise. The same goes for any time you feel dizzy or nauseous. Listening to your body is vital when exercising because it can keep you from pushing yourself beyond your limit. As such, it can reduce the likelihood of hurting yourself in one way or another and enable you to adjust your plans safely.

As you can see, creating a fitness plan for yourself is fairly simple as long as you are aware of your fitness level and goals. The same goes for creating a nutrition plan that works for you. For this, you'll need to understand what your personal nutrition needs are. Since you're now going to be working out regularly, for example, you're going to need to consume 0.8 to 2 grams of protein per pound of your body weight. Otherwise, you won't be able to build any muscle, as you'll recall. This is especially true for nonathletes who are not used to working out.

Likewise, you're going to have to remember your various health conditions as you make your nutrition plan. If you have diabetes or insulin resistance, for instance, that's clearly going to affect which foods you're allowed to eat and what quantities you're allowed to eat them in.

One sound strategy to adopt here might be to speak with either a dietician or a nutritionist before you start putting together your nutrition plan. That way, you can be sure you're doing what's right for you, personally. Every human being has a different constitution, after all, which means that a dietary plan that worked for a friend of yours won't necessarily work for you. Speaking with a nutritionist should also help you grasp what your caloric needs are. How many calories you need per day depends on what your activity levels are. Someone who leads a sedentary lifestyle sitting in their office chair from 7 a.m. to 8 p.m. will need fewer calories than someone who vigorously works out for an hour every day. Likewise, someone who works out vigorously every day won't need as many calories as an Olympic athlete. That's only to be expected. Your nutrition plan, then, will need to take your fitness plan into account if it is to be accurate and good for you.

You can calculate your caloric needs by using one of two equations. If you're a woman, the basal metabolic rate (BMR) formula you need is (NutritionED Contributor, 2022)

Your Activity Level x [[(10 x Your Weight in kg) + (6.25 X Your Height in cm) + (5 x Your Age in Years)] - 161]

If you're a man, then the basal metabolic rate (BMR) formula you need is

Your Activity Level x [[(10 x Your Weight in kg) + (6.25 X Your Height in cm) + (5 x Your Age in Years)] + 5]

What your activity level equals depends on how active a lifestyle you lead:

- If you lead a sedentary lifestyle, your activity level is 1.2.
- If you lead a lightly active lifestyle, your activity level is 1.375.

- If you lead a moderately active lifestyle, your activity level is 1.55.

- If you lead an active lifestyle, your activity level is 1.725.

- If you lead a very active lifestyle, your activity level is 1.9.

In any case, the end result of these equations is officially referred to as your total daily energy expenditure (TDEE). If you mean to gain muscle, then as a rule, you'll have to eat 250 calories more than what's shown in your TDEE. If you mean to shred fat, you will need to eat fewer calories than your TDEE, referred to as eating in a calorie deficit.

Now that you're aware of this fact, you can actually start planning out what you're going to be eating. Obviously, you'll have to look up the calories of the various ingredients you'll be using and the dishes you'll be making with them. There are a great many apps you can use that can help you figure this out quickly and, thus, plan accordingly. Planning your meals using these apps is not only a great way of making sure you abide by your caloric requirements but also of figuring out what you'll be eating in advance. Try to decide on your dishes for the next week at the end of each week. Then, take a look at your fridge and pantry to see which ingredients you're missing. After that, take care of your grocery shopping, and you'll be ready to cook. You can always prepare your meals a day in advance, but it would be more advisable to cook for the whole week or at least do the prep work of your dishes for the coming days. That way, you can pick up speed in the kitchen, which is something you'll appreciate on busy workdays and after you come home from the gym feeling ravenous.

Tracking Progress Effectively

Tracking your fitness progress is a vital part of working out. This is because it helps you see how far you've come, adjust your plan to accommodate your current fitness level, and work toward your fitness goals more easily. So, how exactly can you track your fitness progress? Truthfully, there are several ways for you to do this. One is to keep a fitness journal. A fitness journal is a journal in which you enter your workout start and end times, the number of sets and reps you've done, the weights you used, and the distances you've covered, assuming you're doing an activity like jogging or cycling (Cook, 2021). Furthermore, it's a document where you write down how many calories you've consumed that day, which you'll be aware of thanks to those apps you're using.

Like any journal, a fitness journal should be updated every day. That way, you'll be able to visibly track the daily progress you make. At the same time, you should write down how you feel after each and every one of your workouts. Odds are, you're going to be feeling pretty energized and good. Recording this information might not sound like it's all that important but this data can serve as an important reminder as to why you're doing what you're doing, especially on days when you're feeling more lethargic.

If you don't want to bother with writing in a journal, be it a physical notebook or a digital document, you can always just use a fitness tracker or app of some sort. You have a myriad of options to choose from in this regard, too. MyFitnessPal, which helps you keep track of all sorts of nutritional information, is one. Stronglifts, which serves as a kind of workout log, is another. Still another is FitNotes, which works in much the same way that Stronglifts does, except it factors in your daily activity levels, too. Meanwhile, a Fitbit helps you track the amount of time you spend moving about on any given day, and Jefit is a great tool to use when building your workout plans.

It might be that you dislike apps or are forgetful when it comes to them. Should that be the case, you can always snap workout pictures of yourself in the mirror and try four poses to track progress: front, back, side, and a flex pose. You're not going to notice a huge difference between your first and, say, third photos. However, as time goes by and you accumulate more and more photos, you'll be able to visibly trace your transformation. Seeing plain evidence that you're changing in this regard will be immensely motivating for you. The same can be said for paying attention to how your clothes fit. Has a pair of pants that used to be too tight suddenly started fitting better? Does a particular suit feel looser? Have you realized that you now have to notch your belt a little more tightly now? All of this is clear evidence that your nutrition and training plans are working.

Such evidence, therefore, cannot be ignored, just as the ever-changing figure that appears on the scale cannot be ignored. The one caveat here, of course, is that the scale doesn't always tell the full truth. You see, your weight is something that can fluctuate from day to day, depending on water retention and bowel movements. On a given day, your weight can fluctuate as much as 6 lbs, and at a minimum, it can fluctuate 2 lbs. The scale can also sometimes be deceiving because muscle is more dense than fat. So, you might be losing fat, and the figure on the scale might be staying the same. It might even be increasing slightly. Given that, measuring yourself with a tape measure often yields more accurate results than getting on the scale. For the most accurate results, you should measure your hips, thighs, waist, shoulders, biceps, and neck at the same time of day. You can then record the results in a small notebook. Over time, you'll find that the figures you write down are getting smaller and smaller because muscle is leaner than fat. Hence, it doesn't take up the same amount of room in your body.

By using these figures, you can effectively and accurately keep track of your fitness level. How quickly your fitness level improves, of course, will depend on how quickly you're able to increase your stamina and build muscle. Prioritizing strength training while working out will help with this, as will choosing the kinds of foods you're going to eat with care. You already know that certain kinds of plant-based foods are great for building muscle. But which ones have the highest protein content? What micro- and macronutrient needs do you need to meet in order to build muscles in a healthy way? How can you utilize calorie surpluses and deficits? The answers to all these questions will directly affect the kind of plant-powered plate you design for yourself and how you approach the design process in the first place.

Chapter 3:

Crafting a Plant-Powered Plate

Leading a healthy life is all about what you put into your body. Feed your body the right nutrients, and it will feel energized and work at optimal levels. Feed it the wrong kinds of nutrients, however, and your energy levels will start going down. You'll feel lethargic and unmotivated, which will obviously impede your efforts to work out. You already know that eating a plant-based meal is the ideal way of providing your body with all the nutrients it needs, but what kind of plant-based diet? There are many types to choose from, after all.

A plant-based diet simply means the kind of diet that places emphasis on foods that have been derived from them and prioritizes them in your meals. Fruits and vegetables are obvious examples of such foods, but so are nuts, seeds, whole grains, and oils. Vegetarian and vegan diets are both prime examples of plant-based diets. However, they're not the only ones.

One of the primary characteristics of any plant-based diet is that it simply entails high consumption of plant-based foods. It requires that people consume much lower quantities of saturated fats, fatty or processed meats, refined grains, and salt than they otherwise would. It can include dairy products, dairy alternatives, and seafood, too, though a vegan diet does not.

Of all the plant-based diets, vegetarianism and veganism are probably the best-known ones, especially given how quickly they've been spreading throughout the world over the last decade. As of 2022, approximately 5-8% of the US population considers themselves vegetarians with about 1 million people who do not consume any animal products (*What Percentage of the Population Is Vegetarian?*, 2023). There's a very simple reason that vegetarianism and veganism are the most popular plant-based diets out there, and that's the fact that they are the healthy forms of this type of diet. This is because they make ample room for all the core components of a good plant-based meal.

The Core Components of a Balanced Plant-Based Meal

What are the core components of a balanced, plant-based meal, and how can you make sure you eat enough of them? This might seem like a complicated task, but it's actually quite easy as long as you use the plate method. The plate method is a highly effective strategy that ensures you meet all your nutrient needs. According to this method, your plate should contain three essential food groups, these being

- fruits and vegetables

- grains and starches

- proteins (*The Plate Method*, 2022)

Half your plate should be made up of fruits and vegetables. The remaining half should be divided into two equal portions—one made up of grains and starches while the other is made up of proteins. Vegetables and fruits should take up this much space on your plate because they're packed with essential nutrients and antioxidants, as you've already seen. Meanwhile, grains and starches should equal a quarter of your plate, given the fact that they have a lot of minerals and vitamin B in them. Grains and starches are essentially carbs, which means they can offer you a great deal of energy. While you need this energy, it's important that you don't eat too many carbs; otherwise, you'll be ingesting too many calories, and your blood sugar levels will suddenly start climbing.

As for proteins, these are an important source of vitamins and minerals and are essential for your muscle-building efforts. When you're choosing your protein sources, it's important that you go for things like legumes and tofu over commercialized protein options, such as a fast-food chain's vegan entrees. Otherwise, you'll be letting a lot of unwanted nutrients, like trans fats and saturated fats, into your body, which can be immensely damaging to your health, especially when they're consumed regularly.

There are three other food categories that you should be consuming as part of your plant-based diet. These are fats, dairy or dairy substitutes, and supplements. Fats are an incredibly important part of your diet and should not be excluded from it. Fats play an essential role in your body's ability to absorb vitamins. Without them, the vitamins you ingest with your food would just pass through your digestive system and be expelled through your regular bowel movements. Of course, not all fats are good for you. There are specific kinds you need and specific kinds you should avoid. The kinds of fats you want in your system are ones that come from organic whole foods. Avocados, for example, are a great source of fat, as are nuts and seeds. Homemade peanut butter—the kind without any added sugar and chemicals in it—is one tasty and healthy fat source for you to go with. Food sources that are rich in omega-3 fatty acids, such as flaxseed and hemp seeds, are too.

Aside from fats, you can also incorporate a small amount of dairy products or dairy substitutes (if vegan). You can eat them either as snacks or use them as ingredients in your meals. Since human beings weren't exactly born to consume milk and milk products—this is why lactose intolerance is a thing—going for plant-based dairy alternatives is your best bet. Such alternatives can be a fantastic source of calcium for you, as well as supply you with some additional protein. Calcium is vital for your bone strength and density. Of course, you can get calcium from other plant-based foods as well, such as beans and dark leafy greens. These foods' calcium content, however, will be much lower than that of dairy products and their plant-based substitutes.

One final thing you might want to incorporate into your diet is daily supplements. The kinds of supplements you need to take may differ from those of someone else since every human being's needs are inherently different, as we keep saying. Two that you might want to prioritize, though, are vitamin B12 and vitamin D. This is because these two vitamins aren't found in plant-based foods in large quantities.

Taking these supplements can keep you from experiencing a deficiency of some sort, especially if you've opted for vegetarianism or veganism.

Meeting Macronutrient and Micronutrient Needs

Having discovered what the core components of plant-based meals are, you might be wondering, "Why these food groups, specifically?" Yes, you know that these foods contain certain nutrients that are vital for your health and well-being, but what, precisely, do they have to offer you, and how badly do you really need them?

Answering this question probably requires understanding what nutrients truly are. "Nutrients" is the overarching term used to describe the essential elements that are found in fats, carbs, proteins, vitamins, and minerals. These essential elements can be divided into two separate categories: micronutrients and macronutrients. What exactly is the difference between the two? Well, macronutrients are the main nutrients to be found in the foods you eat. These are nutrients that your body absolutely needs to be able to function and maintain the integrity of its structure. They come from the proteins, carbs, and fats that you consume and can be measured in grams. By counting these grams, you can actually keep track of the amount of macronutrients you're ingesting on a daily basis. In doing so, you can make sure you're not overconsuming or underconsuming them.

The recommended macronutrient ratio for a healthy diet can vary depending on your age, sex, activity level, and overall health goals. However, here are some general guidelines (Espinosa-Salas & Gonzalez-Arias, 2023):

- Carbohydrates: 45-65% of total daily calories

- Protein: 10-35% of total daily calories

- Fat: 20-35% of total daily calories

If you want to optimize fat loss, however, then the guidelines you need to follow are

- Carbohydrates: 10-30% of total daily calories

- Protein: 40-50% of total daily calories

- Fat: 20-30% of total daily calories

Reducing your carbohydrate intake can help control blood sugar levels and promote fat utilization. Higher protein intake can support muscle preservation and satiety during calorie restriction.

As for optimizing muscle growth, the guidelines you have to follow in this case are

- Carbohydrates: 45-65% of total daily calories

- Protein: 15-25% of total daily calories

- Fat: 20-35% of total daily calories.

To optimize muscle growth, it's important to ensure an adequate intake of carbohydrates to provide energy for workouts and protein to support muscle repair and growth.

Count the macronutrients that you're consuming and take a look at how many calories you've ingested today. How much of that has come from carbs? How much of it has come from fats and proteins? If you're under the prescribed amount, then you can stand to increase your macronutrient intake. If, on the other hand, you're over the prescribed limits, then you can stand to take it down a notch or two.

What are micronutrients, then? "Micronutrients" is the catch-all term for vitamins and minerals you consume. They're measured in milligrams. Your body needs smaller quantities of micronutrients than it needs macronutrients. This is because, unlike macronutrients, micronutrients don't supply your body with the energy it needs to function. It does, however, need micronutrients to be able to perform at optimal levels. Without micronutrients, for instance, your body wouldn't be able to properly perform daily tasks like digesting the food you're eating or producing the hormones you need.

Unless we're talking about vitamin B12 and vitamin D, you want to meet all your micronutrient needs through the plant-based whole foods you eat. Luckily, this is easy to do, as long as you maintain a varied diet. Different kinds of vitamins are found in different kinds of fruits and vegetables, after all. You can meet your vitamin B9 needs by eating more asparagus, for example. Meanwhile, you can make sure to consume more vitamin B5 by consuming shitake mushrooms, and you can get more vitamin B6 from potatoes and chickpeas. Meanwhile, you'll find plenty of potassium in lentils and raisins, which is good news because the mineral known as potassium helps with muscle functioning. You can find another mineral, magnesium, in foods like spinach, almonds, and pumpkin seeds too.

Calculating Your Macros and Designing Meals for Muscle Growth and Fat Loss

Counting your macros—that is to say, your protein, carb, and fat intake—is vital if you are to succeed at your muscle-building efforts. As you'll remember, you need to eat 0.8 to 1 gram of protein per body weight in pounds if you want to build muscle. What do fats and carbs have to do with muscle building, though? Isn't this all about proteins? Actually, it's not. Carbs and fats play just as important a role in muscle building as proteins do.

Fats get a bad rep for the most part, but they're essential for your body's health and well-being since they help it to absorb the vitamins you ingest. Obviously, having too many fat deposits is a bad thing, but having a low fat intake can be highly problematic, too. If your fat intake is below the required levels, your hormonal functions will be repressed, which will mean all sorts of health problems for you. You can avoid this by eating 0.3 grams of fat per pound of your body weight. As for carbs, they're your body's main energy source. Not eating enough carbs means not having enough energy to function, much less exercise. To avoid this, you should aim for a range of 0.60 grams to 1 gram of carbs per pound of body weight. To shred fat, stick to the lower number in the range; to add muscle, choose the higher range. This, right here, is part of the reason why half of your plate is made up of fruits and vegetables in the plate method.

This obviously doesn't include fiber. While fiber is a kind of carb that exists in abundance in fruits and vegetables, it cannot be fully digested in your body. Hence, it's often expelled from it via your digestive tract. This doesn't make fiber useless, though. On the contrary, fiber is essential for your gut health since it helps the good bacteria in your gut to absorb the nutrients you eat. At the same time, it slows down how quickly your blood sugar levels rise and improves your heart health, among many other things. Fiber also tends to slow down digestion. This is a good thing. So, if you want to have enough energy to work out, you shouldn't eat high-fiber foods immediately before your workouts.

Now that you know what the exact amounts of macronutrients you need to consume are, all that's left is for you to calculate the macros in your meals. You can do this using an app or pen and paper. You'll need to measure the dry ingredients you'll be cooking with, though, so that you can get as accurate a result as humanly possible. A scale will be optimal for this. Once you've measured your ingredients, you can enter them into your app or notebook and keep track of your macros there. Alternatively, you can use the hand method. Though the hand method will be a little more ballpark than actually counting macros is, it is no less accurate for it. The method is fairly simple, too. It states that

- the dry protein you eat should be no bigger than your palm

- the dry carbs you eat shouldn't exceed the size of your four fingers put together

- the fat you consume shouldn't be more than the size of your palm

While you generally want to physically count the macros you eat, the hand method can save you a lot of trouble if you're in a rush, traveling, or just having a hectic day. It can successfully support your efforts to design meals that will support both your weight loss and your muscle gain (English, 2020). Of course, while you're counting your macros, you'll have to pay close attention to where you're getting them from. Obviously, you'll be favoring plant-based foods, but which ones will be best for your macronutrient needs? More specifically, which plant-based foods will be ideal to meet your protein needs, and which combinations will be able to ensure that you get all the amino acids your body requires into your system?

Chapter 4:

Plant Protein Mastery

By now, it should be obvious that there are a staggering number of plant proteins out there for you to choose from. It should also be obvious that you can't just eat one type of plant protein all the time and call it a day. Do that, and you'll be denying your body some very essential amino acids. As you know, proteins are made up of amino acids, and there are 20 different kinds of amino acids in all. Of these, your body absolutely needs nine very specific ones because it is unable to produce them on its own. It can, however, produce the remaining amino acids by itself. So, those amino acids aren't considered "essential," but consuming more of them can most certainly be helpful.

The nine amino acids that are considered to be must-haves for the health, well-being, and overall functioning of your body are

- histidine
- isoleucine
- leucine
- lysine
- methionine
- phenylalanine
- threonine
- tryptophan

- valine (National Research Council (US) Subcommittee on the Tenth Edition of the Recommended Dietary Allowances, 1989)

Know which plant proteins contain which of these amino acids, and you'll be able to plan meals that can effectively support both your health and your efforts to keep building muscles.

Exploring Diverse Plant-Based Protein Sources

The first plant-based protein you need to add to your diet, if you can, is a rather unexpected one: seitan (Petre & Ajmera, 2022). Seitan is quite popular among people who've adopted plant-based diets, especially vegetarianism or veganism, and for good reason. Aside from being quite healthy, texturally and taste-wise, it closely resembles meat. Seitan is essentially made from gluten, which is a type of protein that can be found in wheat. 3.5 ounces of seitan contains roughly 25 grams of protein. That's a lot, no matter which way you cut it. Crucially, seitan contains all nine of the essential amino acids that you need. In addition to that, it has plenty of selenium to offer you and also serves as a decent source of calcium, phosphorus, and iron. The one downside to seitan is that, given what it's made of, it's not a good option for people with gluten allergies to eat.

For those who cannot eat seitan, tofu, tempeh, or even edamame could be great alternatives to consider. These three food items may sound like they're entirely different from one another, but they're all made of soybeans, which are rich in protein. Tofu, for example, is made from soybean curds that have been pressed together. Tempeh, on the other hand, is made from cooked, then slightly fermented soybeans, whereas edamame is just immature soybeans that have been harvested early. Like seitan, tofu contains the nine essential amino acids you need, as do tempeh and edamame. Unlike its compatriots, tofu doesn't have much of a taste. Thus, it readily absorbs the flavors of whatever it's cooked with, making it extremely versatile. Meanwhile, tempeh retains a more nutty flavor, whereas edamame tastes sweet, even a little grassy. Like their tastes, there are some differences in their nutritional profiles, too. Tempeh, for instance, is very rich in vitamin B, various probiotics, phosphorus, and magnesium. Edamame, on the other hand, is rich in fiber, folates, and vitamin K.

If those foods of the soybean variety don't really suit your tastes, you can always go for lentils. Lentils offer you 18 grams of protein per cup and have all nine essential amino acids, but their tryptophan and methionine supplies are pretty limited. Aside from that, lentils are rich in fiber. In fact, they have a very specific kind of fiber in them that supports the healthy bacteria in your gut. They're rich in folates, iron, and manganese, too, along with antioxidants, which makes them a powerhouse of a food group.

Lentils are a member of the legume family. The same goes for beans, which are yet another great source of protein. There are all kinds of different beans you can enjoy, like pinto beans, cannellini, and black beans. Unlike the other plant-based proteins we've discussed so far, beans don't have all nine essential amino acids in them. They only have some, and which ones they have depends on which type of bean you're eating. Proteins that don't have all essential amino acids in them are known as incomplete proteins, which is what beans are. Most bean types have about 15 grams of protein in them per cup. They're generally rich in fiber, phosphorus, folate, iron, potassium, manganese, as well as carbs. Hence, they're a good nutritional powerhouse, too, as well as a good source of energy for you. They come with the typical benefits that accompany most legumes, such as helping to reduce belly fat, lower cholesterol levels, and lower blood sugar levels.

Seeds can be an excellent source of protein, too. Of these, one kind of seed that immediately catches the eye is hemp seeds. Unlike beans, hemp seeds do have all nine essential amino acids in them. Three tablespoons of hempseed contain as much as 9 grams of protein. On top of that, they contain an abundance of magnesium, zinc, selenium, omega-3 fatty acids, omega-6 fatty acids, and calcium.

Green peas are another member of the legume family that have all nine essential amino acids within them. A cup of green peas has 9 grams of protein in it. All this means that pea protein, which is a meat alternative you can buy and eat, is a great amino acid source for you. It further means that you can eat spoonfuls of peas to your heart's content to meet your protein needs. Peas contain a lot more than proteins, though. Their fiber, folate, thiamine, vitamin A, vitamin C, vitamin K, and manganese levels are through the roof.

Another rather unexpected source of protein to consider is nutritional yeast. Sold in yellow powder format, this is a type of deactivated yeast. It has all nine essential amino acids in it and tastes a bit like cheese. You can get 8 grams of protein from half an ounce of nutritional yeast, as well as a lot of copper, manganese, zinc, magnesium, and varieties of vitamin B. In fact, vitamin B12 can be found in abundance in nutritional yeast, unlike most plant-based foods. This only goes for fortified yeast, though. So, you must always check what type of yeast you're getting before you head to the checkout counter.

Two protein sources that you might not have ever heard of are teff and spelt. Teff and spelt are both ancient grains. Spelt is actually a type of wheat. It has gluten, which means that it should not be eaten by those who are allergic to gluten. Teff, on the other hand, is made from grass. Thus, it's devoid of gluten and perfect for people with gluten allergies. A cooked cup of spelt or teff has 10 to 11 grams of protein in it, which is great since they both harbor all nine essential amino acid types. Additionally, they have high levels of fiber, complex carbs, iron, magnesium, manganese, and plenty of vitamins.

Then there's spirulina, an ingredient that has been getting more and more attention of late. Spirulina is very nutritionally rich, but it doesn't contain all nine essential amino acids. Still, the ones it does have, it has in abundance. In addition to all sorts of nutrients, spirulina has a pigment called phycocyanin. This pigment is a powerful antioxidant that has both anti-inflammatory and anticancer properties. Hence, it's definitely a good ingredient to add to the menu.

Quinoa and amaranth are also great options to consider, as they're both ancient, gluten-free grains that are packed with protein. Both contain the nine essential amino acids, and a single cup of either will have 8-9 grams of protein in it. They're good complex carb, fiber, and mineral sources to boot.

Like tofu, soy milk is a product that's made from soybeans, and it's one you should add to your shopping list if you can, especially if you're looking for good milk alternatives. As a soybean product, it contains all essential amino acids, and a single cup will offer you 6 grams of protein. Not only that, but it'll introduce plenty of calcium and vitamin D to your system. The one thing to remember when you're getting soy milk is to make sure it doesn't have any added sugar in it. As a rule, unsweetened varieties are best for milk alternatives. This goes just as much for oat milk as it does for soy milk.

Oat milk and oats, by extension, are great protein sources in and of themselves. There are 5 grams of protein in just half a cup of oats, as well as 4 grams of fiber. The one caveat about oats is that they don't have all essential amino acids in them, making them an incomplete protein. The same, however, cannot be said about wild rice, which is an infinitely better option than other types of rice. This is because wild rice has 1.5 times the protein content than they do. To get a little more specific, a cup of wild rice has about 7 grams of protein. Since wild rice isn't stripped of its bran, it has more fiber, vitamins, and minerals to offer you, too.

To go back to seeds for a moment, chia seeds are a great protein source for you. As a complete protein, chia seeds have 5 grams of protein for every 28 grams. They're very nutritionally rich and can absorb a lot of water, which means they can help you to stay hydrated. Nuts don't have the same absorbent quality, but that doesn't mean they're any less of a protein source for you. They have high nutrition content, as well as a wide variety of amino acids to offer you, depending on what kind of nuts or nut butter you're eating. Ideally, you want to eat nuts raw, as opposed to roasted or blanched, since those procedures can damage their nutritional profile. If you're having some kind of nut butter, making some at home or purchasing a jar that's sugar and chemical free would be best.

On top of all this, there are a number of protein-rich fruits and vegetables you can add to your grocery list. Admittedly, some of these contain more proteins than others, and not all of them are complete proteins. The vegetables that have the highest protein content, however, are

- Brussels sprouts
- potatoes and sweet potatoes

- broccoli

- spinach

- asparagus

- artichokes

Typically speaking, these vegetables have about 4 to 5 grams of protein per single, cooked cup. As for fruits, the ones with the highest protein content are

- blackberries

- nectarines

- bananas

- guava

Fruits have a lower protein content than vegetables. The ones listed here, for instance, usually have between 2 and 4 grams of protein per cup in them. Nonetheless, eating more of them will not only increase your protein intake but also ensure you meet all your nutritional needs.

Proper Timing and Quantity of Protein Intake

Choosing the kinds of protein you eat is just one part of meeting your protein requirements while building muscle. For optimal results, you're going to have to consider two additional things: when you're going to eat your protein and how much of it you're going to eat per day. These two things may not sound all that important, especially that first one, but they actually play a crucial role in the muscle-building process. For instance, studies show that the best time to eat more protein is in the morning, with your breakfast, if you want to build muscle (Aoyama et al., 2021). The reason for this has to do with the way in which your body metabolizes the different kinds of macronutrients you consume. Your body is able to digest protein quickly when you have it in the morning. People who eat protein for breakfast develop muscle more quickly, and the size of their muscles ultimately ends up being bigger than those who don't.

Breakfast isn't the only time you should be eating protein, though. If you want to build muscle, then you need to have some 15 minutes to 2 hours after your workout session (Raman, 2018). This window of time, known as the anabolic window, is considered by many to be the perfect time to ingest protein. This makes sense when you think about it. When you work out, microtears form on your muscles, as you know. Your body gets to work repairing those and uses the amino acids found in proteins to do so. Giving your body protein up to 2 hours after your workout session means giving it more amino acids to work with. Just as a building cannot the built without enough cement blocks, your muscles can't be built without enough amino acids.

As for how much protein you should be eating, the answer to this question is partly related to how old you are. If you're over 30 years old, then your body will start losing 3-8% of its muscle mass every decade. You can prevent this by building more muscle, which means both working out and eating more protein. Hence, if you're over 30 years old, you should be eating 25-30 grams of protein per meal. This will amount to 1.2-2 grams of protein per 0.54 to 0.9 pounds of your body weight every day. In other words, it'll mean between 81 and 136 grams of protein for your average 150-pound adult (Satrazemis, 2022).

Combining Proteins for Different Amino Acid Options

While it's true that there are a lot of plant-based proteins that have the nine essential amino acids you need, it's also true that they have them in different quantities. In addition to that, some don't have all the amino acids you need. If you want to ensure you're getting all the amino acids you need, you have to combine your plant-based proteins in different ways. To that end, some of the best protein combos you can go for are

- nut butter, such as peanut butter, on a slice of whole wheat toast

- beans and wild rice or other kinds of rice

- hummus—which is made from chickpeas, a legume—and whole wheat pita chips

- lentil soup with a whole grain bread roll to dip into it

- lentil and barley soup

- salad made with spinach leaves, sunflower seeds, and chickpeas

- bean soup and crackers

- peas and whole wheat pasta

- lentils with a handful of almonds tossed in while cooking (*How to Eat Complete Proteins in Vegetarian and Vegan Diets*, 2022)

Chapter 5:

Fueling Your Workouts: Pre-, Intra-, and Postnutrition

Working out takes a lot of energy out of you. This holds true no matter what sports activity you're engaging in, be it hitting the gym, playing team sports, going swimming, or something else. Given that, you have to make sure to keep your energy levels up by providing your body with all the fuel that it needs. This means eating specific kinds of foods for a set period before you start working out. If your workouts are particularly long or if you're playing a team sport of some sort, then it also means snacking during break times. There's a reason why professional basketball players and the like can be seen munching on one thing or another during timeouts. Likewise, it means eating plenty of food after you're done working out. As you've seen, you need to eat some sort of protein up to two hours after you've finished with your workout if you want to build more muscle. What precisely should you be eating before, during, and after your workouts, though? How much should you be eating during those specific periods, for that matter?

Energizing Your Sessions with Smart, Preworkout Meals

So, you've decided on your workout schedule and aim to stick loyally to it. Now, you just have to start hitting the gym at your scheduled times, right? Yes, but before then, you need to plan out what meals you'll be eating before starting your workout. As a rule, you don't want to eat anything right before your workout. Doing so is a decidedly bad idea because it can cause you to develop a cramp. It can also make you nauseous. Alternatively, the food you've ingested may feel too heavy for you to keep functioning. Experts recommend that you eat a full meal three hours before you work out (Head, 2021). You can have a light snack an hour before you work out, too. Whatever snack you go with must be something that has low levels of fat, mid levels of protein, and higher carb levels. A banana with some peanut butter is a good example of a snack that fits this description. So is a rice cake.

How about your preworkout meal? What type of preworkout meal you're going to go with will depend on what kind of activity you'll be doing. Say that you decide to add High Intensity Interval Training (HIIT). True to their name, HIIT workouts are quite intense. Thus, they require you to have a lot of energy. Hence, you will need to eat proteins and carbs that release really quickly in your body. Scrambled eggs on rye toast is a good example of this if eggs are included in your chosen diet plan. So is whole grain pasta with tomato sauce or even whole grain toast with a layer of peanut butter on it.

What if you're doing cardio, like going running, instead? In that case, you will need food that's light on the stomach but can give you plenty of carbs to work or, rather, work out with. A bowl of oatmeal with some banana slices over it would fit the bill very nicely, especially for long runs. For shorter runs, four rice cakes with honey, depending on your diet, could be really good, especially since the carbs and sugar you get with those will give you the burst of energy you need to start sprinting. The key thing to remember when choosing food before you go on a run is that said food cannot be high in fiber. As useful as it is, high fiber can easily lead to bloating while running, and this can, in turn, upset your stomach, causing you to quit your workout session halfway through.

Another cardio exercise you might be doing is cycling or going to a spin class. A spin class is a high-intensity environment where you can burn as much as 400 to 600 calories in one go. Classes last 45 minutes on average, so you can imagine how heavy a workout you'll be in for. You can also imagine just how much energy you'll need to get through your class. Given that, you'll need to eat a decent meal with enough carbs in it to sustain you. One example of such a meal might be a baked sweet potato topped with some guacamole with tomato chunks in it. You could also try a salad made with baby spinach leaves, sunflower seeds, olive oil, and pine nuts, or even a fresh smoothie made with some delicious high-protein fruits.

Alternatively, you might be doing something that requires a bit more flexibility, like yoga, Pilates, or barre. Since these kinds of exercises are slower and steadier, especially compared to cardio exercises like running, you don't need to eat a full meal to be able to stock up on energy. Instead, it would be better to go with a light snack, one that can keep your blood sugar levels from rising and crashing suddenly. If you are going to have a meal, then slower-releasing carbs and proteins are best. Carrots and hummus, Greek yogurt or dairy-free yogurt with a dash of cinnamon and some berries sprinkled on top, or an oat cake topped with a boiled egg might be good options to consider.

Of course, there's always strength training, which is likely what you'll be doing to build muscle. This can entail training using your own body weight or lifting bars and weights. Whatever type of strength training you're engaged in, you'll need to consume a moderate serving of protein in your preworkout meal. Your meal can also include carbs that are easy to digest, like low-fiber fruits or vegetables. This isn't just because protein promotes muscle growth but also because it reduces the likelihood that you'll feel hungry while working out.

What if you want to combine strength training with cardio? Doing a cardio-weight training circuit might not leave you as exhausted as a HIIT training session might, but it will still be pretty intense. Hence, you'll need lots of energy to sustain you. A meal like a small serving of seitan and guacamole could be just what the doctor ordered with such workouts. For snacks, a handful of mixed nuts is always a good option to consider, as are a couple of squares of dark chocolate, surprisingly enough. Whatever snacks you go for here must be high fat—though said fats must be healthy fats, not unhealthy ones like trans fats—and high protein. This won't just keep your energy levels up, but it'll also increase the production of hormones like dopamine in your brain, making you feel better and increasing both your dedication and focus in the process.

Last but not least, you might be interested in going swimming. While swimming is primarily a cardio exercise, it does have a resistance element to it since you're going up against water resistance with every kick and stroke. A protein-based meal is ideal for this type of exercise. Some leafy greens coupled with an avocado and scrambled eggs immediately come to mind here. So do whole grain oatcakes with avocado or homemade breakfast bars made with mashed bananas, chopped hazelnuts and almonds, and shredded carrots.

Navigating Intraworkout Nutrition

Say that you found yourself getting a little peckish midworkout. What are you supposed to do, ignore your hunger pangs and keep going? Actually, you're not. Instead, you're supposed to have some snacks on hand that you can turn to when you take a break. Having an intraworkout snack—not a meal, mind you—is important because it can ensure your energy levels stay high and consistent. In other words, it can keep your blood sugar level steady and make sure you don't run out of fuel and energy midway through your workout. Of course, for this to be the case, you need to choose your snacks wisely. You don't want to eat something that's going to be too difficult to digest, making you feel like your food is trying to climb its way back up your throat. You also don't want to eat something too light, resulting in your blood sugar levels suddenly crashing, making you feel dizzy and nauseous, and causing your hands to start shaking.

So, which plant-based foods fit this description? First, there's bananas. Bananas are a great snack for workouts that last longer than an hour (*10 Mid-Workout Snacks to Sustain Performance*, 2021). One reason for this is that they are very easy to digest. Another is that, as carbs, they serve as quick sources of energy, giving you a much-needed boost. As an added bonus, bananas are packed with potassium, which is a mineral that helps relieve physical stress in your muscles and body.

Bananas aren't your only fruit option as far as snacks are concerned. Far from it. In fact, watery fruits make for some of the best snacks possible. Orange and cantaloupe slices are among such fruits, and they can effectively help you keep your performance and energy levels high.

Watery fruits, you see, are high in natural sugars and vitamins. Your body ends up using its sugar and vitamin stores while you're working out. By eating watery fruits, you get to replenish them. Not only that, but watery fruits obviously have a high water content. By eating them, you actually prevent dehydration. Of course, you should be regularly drinking water throughout your training session regardless, but watery fruits will still be of help to you.

Interestingly enough, dehydrated, that is to say, dried fruits can make for great workout snacks, too. Dried fruits tend to be quite light, as well as bursting with both vitamins and minerals. So they can replenish your body's stores very quickly. They won't, however, slow down your digestive processes since they're low in fiber. This will keep you from expending any additional and, thus, unnecessary energy on digesting what you eat. However, like with most things, there's one caveat to consider where dried fruits are concerned, and that's that sometimes they're packed with added sugar. Therefore, you must always check the nutritional information on the packaging of whichever dried fruits you get.

Protein shakes, which you'll have to prepare in advance, are a great snack option too. A good protein shake can sustain you through long workouts. The protein in it, which will come in the form of protein powder and protein-rich fruits, will aid with muscle recovery while you work out. At the same time, it'll keep your energy levels high. The key to remember here is to choose a kind of protein powder that's fast absorbing. That way, it'll make it through your digestive system quicker and help your muscles repair themselves that much faster.

You already know that nut butters are great plant-based foods to enjoy, but did you know that sunflower butter is an especially good option as a midworkout snack? Like most nuts and seeds, sunflowers have very high protein levels. The main difference from other seeds is that it has an especially high vitamin content. This makes it ideal as a snack, particularly when it's spread over some green apple slices or with some carrot or celery sticks dipped into it.

A final, rather surprising snack you might want to consider is pretzels. Pretzels are clearly very rich in carbs and salt. You need carbs to replenish your energy levels, but you need to raise your salt levels back up to par, too. This is because you end up losing a lot of salt when you sweat, which you inevitably will do when working out. That means losing plenty of electrolytes, which are vital for your body's ability to function properly. The advantage of replenishing your energy and electrolyte levels with pretzels is that they're very light. So, they won't make you feel stuffed or queasy, thereby getting in the way of your workout. A handful of pretzels can do wonders for you while you're exercising, as long as you remember to pack them.

Optimizing Recovery with Postworkout Meals

Just as you need to make sure you've eaten before you work out, you need to have a proper meal after you're done, too. Since you will have spent plenty of energy while exercising, you're going to have to eat pretty quickly once you're done. To be specific, you're going to want to eat a meal that contains plenty of carbs, as well as protein, at most two hours after your training session has concluded. If you are unable to eat a full meal during that time, you should at least eat a high-protein and carb snack.

As far as postworkout snacks go, a plant-based protein drink like the kind you had during your workout, yogurt with some fruit, or a peanut butter and jam sandwich on whole grain toast are grand ideas. You should try to eat your snacks or, ideally, your meal about 30 minutes after your training session has ended if you can. In the meantime, you might start preparing your meals. Some choice dishes for you to make for yourself might be

- a Buddha bowl
- pasta with lentil Bolognese sauce
- lentil spinach curry with rice
- tofu quiche
- a cous cous bowl with crispy tofu

- chickpea frittata
- three bean soup
- red lentil dahl
- a sweet potato bowl

Whatever dish you choose to prepare, there'll be one rule you'll need to abide by, assuming you want to keep building muscle, and that's to follow a 4:1 carb to protein ratio. This way, you'll be able to replenish all your energy and your amino acid levels, giving your body everything it needs to repair the microtears in your muscles. In addition to that, you need to include ingredients that can help bring inflammation down throughout your body. Ingredients that can do that are ones that are rich in antioxidants, as you know, and omega-3 fatty acids. Having said that, you don't want your postworkout meals to be too fat heavy since fats slow down the digestion process.

Chapter 6:

The Role of Carbohydrates in Muscle Building and Fat Loss

By now, it's abundantly clear that you need to eat protein to build muscle, but what about carbs? What role do they play in weight loss and muscle gain? Are there any specific kinds of carbs you should be eating? Obviously, carbs are your primary source of energy. That means you're going to have to eat some, especially if you're going to be working out. Otherwise, your body won't have enough energy to repair your muscles and keep itself fit and healthy. Eating carbs can actually prevent muscle loss. When you consume the amount of carbs you are required to eat per day, you give your body the ability to maintain the muscle mass it already possesses. Without carbs, your body simply won't have enough energy to resume its normal functions properly (Meyer, 2023). Hence, the microtears on your muscles will remain unrepaired. Over time, your damaged muscles will start breaking down, and they'll be converted to energy for your body to use. Hence, you'll lose muscle mass.

Alternatively, not eating enough carbs can cause your muscle recovery process to slow down. Lacking in energy, your body will take longer to repair the microtears over your muscles. This will only increase the soreness you feel after your workouts, as well as how long you feel it. It will increase your general fatigue, too. You can prevent all this from happening, though, by eating 0.6 to 2 grams of carbs per kilogram of body weight per day. This will not only improve your energy levels significantly but also prevent hypertrophy, that is to say, loss of muscle mass. Eating a serving of carbs about an hour before strength training sessions will do the same, as will eating carbs immediately after your workout and two to three hours after you're done exercising.

Carbohydrates as Performance Fuel

Clearly, then, carbs are one of the best things for you to eat before, during, and after your training sessions. The benefits that carbs have to offer you as a fuel source become especially evident in workouts that last longer than an hour. Scientists have known since about the 1930s that your overall performance level can be significantly improved by increasing the amount of carbs you include in your daily diet. To understand the reason behind this, you must first grasp how carbs are stored in your body.

When you eat carbs, what you've consumed gets turned into a substance called glycogen. We say that carbs are your fuel source, but really, it's glycogen that powers your cells, organs, systems, and muscles. When you eat an excess of carbs, you end up with an excess of glycogen. That excess glycogen is then stored across your body as fuel deposits, so to speak. When you work out, you start burning through those fuel deposits. If you work out once in a blue moon, then, obviously, you're not going to run out of your deposits. If you're working out regularly, however, you are eventually going to burn through them. In other words, you're going to start losing fat and, thus, losing weight.

While losing weight can be a good thing, you need and want to replenish the energy deposits you're losing. The only way to do that, at the end of the day, is to eat more carbs so that they can be turned into glycogen and power your muscles. Do that, and not only will you improve your performance levels—there's a marked difference between how well an energized and exhausted athlete can perform, after all—but you'll also delay the onset of fatigue.

This only goes for complex carbs, though. Complex carbs are decidedly different from simple carbs. Complex carbs are considered "complex" because they contain a lot of nutrients. They help you to keep your blood sugar (glucose) levels steady and keep you fuller after you're done eating a meal or having a snack. Meanwhile, simple carbs do the exact opposite of this. Found in milk, beverages that have been sweetened with sugar or artificial sweeteners, candies, baked goods, and other such foods and ingredients, simple carbs raise your blood sugar levels very quickly. They lower your blood sugar levels pretty quickly, too, causing you to experience a crash every once in a while.

Given that, simple carbs are typically best avoided. This doesn't mean you can't ever eat anything with simple carbs in them. It just means that it has to be in more moderate quantities and more occasionally. In fact, if you're a professional athlete, you're most definitely going to have to make simple carbs a part of your diet, just as complex carbs will be a part of it. This is because achieving the high energy levels you need to be able to perform at optimal levels will be next to impossible without them.

Which complex carbs should you specifically go for then? For that matter, which plant-based carbs should absolutely be made a part of your diet, and which ones should be enjoyed in moderation? Truthfully, the carbs in a plant-based diet aren't all that different from a meat-based diet, at least not if you are maintaining a healthy diet in the first place. Carbs don't just mean bread and rice, after all. They include things like fruits and vegetables, which do have high carb levels. Some of the best fruits and vegetables for you to add to your grocery list are

- barley, which has 135 grams of carbs per cup

- brown rice, which has 45 grams of carbs per cup

- fruits like apples, bananas, berries, and pears, which have 47 grams of carbs per cup

- nonstarchy vegetables like asparagus, broccoli, and peppers, which have 6 grams of carbs per half cup

- starchy vegetables such as potatoes, peas, and corn, which have 20 grams of carbs per half a cup

- sweet potatoes, which have 27 grams of carbs per cup

- whole grain bread, which has 12 grams of carbs per slice

- whole grain pasta, which has 37 grams of carbs per cup (*Vegan Bodybuilding Meal Plan: Plant-Based Muscle Gain*, 2022)

Having said that, some carbs are better able to support your efforts to build muscle than others, and not all of them are complex carbs. Take white rice, for instance. White rice gets a bit of a bad rep since it raises your blood sugar levels pretty quickly. Yet, this doesn't change the fact that it's considered one of the best carbs out there for bodybuilding. This is both because white rice is very easy to digest and because it has a rather bland taste. 100 grams of cooked rice will have about 28.5 grams of carbs in it, which is a lot of energy for you to take advantage of when you think about it (D. J. Sautter, 2023). If you're worried about how white rice will affect your blood sugar levels, you can always go with brown rice, which is higher in fiber and certain micronutrients. In either case, you'll be providing your body with plenty of fuel to work with when you hit the gym.

Like white rice, pasta also has a pretty bad rep, but again, it's actually really good for your muscle-building purposes. This doesn't mean you can eat a whole pot of pasta in one sitting, of course, but you can enjoy a serving of it. Pasta is highly palatable, and it's this very fact that makes it a good choice for you. Since it has 31 grams of carbs per 100 grams of cooked product, it has a lot of energy to offer you. The same goes for both regular and sweet potatoes, which can offer you about 20.1 grams of carbs per 100 grams of cooked product. Both regular and sweet potatoes are easy to digest and very easy for your body to absorb. Hence, they get converted to fuel very easily, supporting your efforts to keep working out and delaying fatigue in the process. Should you choose to have potatoes with their skin still on—which you should—you'll be consuming a lot of folates and phosphates, too, which are both nutrients that your body needs.

Then there's oats, which give you plenty of delicious breakfast options, as you may well know. Oats have 12 grams of carbs per every cooked 100 grams. While that may seem like it's not a lot, at least not in comparison to white rice, it's actually a good boost of energy. What's more, oats are a great source of nutrients, including protein—of all things—and fiber. Hence, they're a vital ingredient for you to consider.

The same can be said of ripe bananas. Bananas make for great snacks, as you've already seen. The key to remember with bananas is that they need to be ripe for you to eat. Unripe bananas, you see, have something called resistant starch in them. This is an undigestible product that your body will eventually expel. As bananas ripen, though, that undigestible product will turn into readily available and digestible carbs. Your body will then be able to quickly absorb those carbs, convert them to energy, and put them to good use.

Certain foods that are known for their protein content also contain a decent amount of carbs. Lentils are a great example of this. Lentils have about 20 grams of carbs per 100 grams of cooked product in them. The carbs that they contain are largely seen as the ideal kind for weight loss and muscle gain because they offer a mix of proteins and carbs. Lentils also feature a broad range of micronutrients, including fiber. Making them a part of your pre- or postworkout meals, then, is an exceptionally good idea.

Finally, there's polenta, which is a very easy-to-use ingredient, given its neutral taste. It has 18.1 grams of carbs per 100 grams of cooked product and offers plenty of protein, much in the same way that lentils do. Thus, they, too, are a phenomenal ingredient to consider for bulking up.

Tailoring Carb Intake to Your Fitness Goals

Generally speaking, you need to eat 0.6 to 2 grams of carbs per pound of body weight per day but that's more of a general rule. This is because the carb requirements of, say, a professional football player are going to be very different from that of someone who just does Pilates twice a week. Like with your caloric needs, the amount of carbs your body needs then depends on your activity level. So, if

- your activity level is very light, meaning you either engage in skill-based activities or do low-intensity exercises, then you'll only need 0.5 to 1 gram of carbs per pound of body weight.

- your activity level is light, meaning you exercise about an hour per day, you'll need 0.7 to 1.5 grams of carbs per pound of body weight.

- your activity level is high, meaning you have an endurance program where you do moderate to high-intensity exercises between 1 and 3 hours per day, you're going to need 1-2 grams of carbs per pound of body weight.

- your activity level is very high, meaning you exercise more than 4-5 hours per day and do moderate- to high-intensity level exercises during that time period, the way a professional athlete would, then you'll need 1 to 2.2 grams of carbs per pound of body weight (Wood, 2020).

What if you don't want to count your carbs or are largely unable to for whatever reason? In that case, you can follow the percentage rules. The percentage rules are pretty simple. If you're not working out at all and simply need to generate enough energy to go about your day-to-day life and activities, then your diet needs to be 40% carbs, 30% protein, and 30% fats. If, on the other hand, you are trying to build muscle and are working out to that end, then your diet needs to be 30% carbs, 40% protein, and 30% fats. How about losing weight, as opposed to building muscle? For this, you'll need your diet to be 50% carbs, 25% protein, and 25% fat (*Unlocking the Power of Macronutrient Ratios*, 2023). Your macronutrient ratios vary depending on your overall goal.

Balancing Carbs to Prevent Fat Gain

As you can see, no matter what your fitness goals are, there is no healthy diet in which you need to cut carbs out of your life entirely. Doing so would, in fact, be very detrimental to your health. If you are worried about your carb intake, then one thing you could do is try carb cycling. Carb cycling is a method of adjusting your carb intake by cycling the different carbs you eat over a period of time to either maintain your current shape or lose fat (Mawer, 2017). Carb cycling can be done on a daily, weekly, or even monthly basis, and it can be done in a variety of different ways. One of them is to reduce your carb intake initially and then add them back in, one by one, when you start trying to build muscle. This methodology has proven to be pretty effective for improving your performance levels or bodybuilding.

Another carb cycling method is to increase your carb intake on days when you will be training and exercising and reduce it on days when you will be resting, thereby meeting your body's daily energy needs. Still another is to tailor your carb intake based on the level or intensity of your training sessions. The more intense a training session is or the longer it lasts, the more carbs you should be consuming to keep your energy levels up. The less intense your workouts are or the shorter they last, the fewer carbs you need to eat. That way, you meet your required energy levels at all times.

The majority of individuals who are using carb cycling to lose weight give themselves two low-carb days, two moderate-carb days, and two high-carb days. Of course, high carb typically translates to low fat. That means that they lower their fat intake on high-carb days and up it on low-carb ones. The reason for this has to do with your body's relationship with fats, as well as with carbs. Carbs get converted to energy, as you already know, but whatever energy you don't expend gets stored in your body as fat deposits. Eat an excess of carbs and fats when you don't have anywhere to spend all the energy you're getting, and you're bound to end up with an excess. In other words, you're bound to gain fat rather than muscle. Should you cut fats out of your diet, then? Not at all. In fact, cutting fats out of your diet could have some severe health repercussions for you, just as cutting carbs would, just in different ways. How, precisely, might cutting fats impact your diet, and why do you need them in the first place?

Chapter 7:

Embracing Healthy Fats

Like carbs, dietary fats often get a bad rep. There's this ever-persistent idea that you need to cut fats entirely out of your diet to lose weight and build muscle. Nothing, however, can be farther from the truth. Not only do you not need to cut fats from your diet, but you cannot afford to, as fats play a vital role in your health and overall well-being. This is because of several reasons. First, healthy dietary fats support the growth and development of your body. Second, fats help your body to absorb essential nutrients, such as vitamins, keeping them from being expelled from your body. They protect the integrity of your cell membranes, keeping them from dissolving. On top of that, they keep your organs warm and provide them with cushioning. They even play a part in the production of various hormones.

This only goes for healthy kinds of fats, though. There are also unhealthy kinds, which you should avoid as much as possible. There are four types of fats out there on the whole:

- polyunsaturated fats

- monounsaturated fats

- saturated fats

- trans fats

Of these, it's the polyunsaturated and monounsaturated fats that can be considered healthy. Meanwhile, saturated fats and trans fats are ones that are unhealthy for you. Saturated fats, you see, can cause your bad cholesterol levels to rise quickly. They can clog your arteries, thereby the blood flow to your heart. These two things can lead to a variety of heart diseases, including strokes and heart attacks. Saturated fats can be found in high-fat dairy, red meat, and poultry. They can even be found in some liquid-form vegetable oils, such as palm oil. Given the health risks that saturated fats entail, experts agree that your intake of them should be limited to 6% of your daily caloric intake at most.

Then there are trans fats, which are what products like margarine contain. Trans fats are vegetable oils that have been heated up using a special process known as hydrogenation, thereby turning them into solid, spreadable food products. They're often used in baked goods, processed foods, and processed and packaged snacks. If you can, you should eliminate trans fats from your diet entirely. If that's not a possibility, then you should limit your intake of them as much as humanly possible. That way, you can prevent them from clogging your arteries and causing some major heart problems for you down the line.

The Importance of Essential Fatty Acids

It needs to be stressed here that it's only unhealthy fats like saturated fats and trans fats that are bad for you, not healthy ones like polyunsaturated and monosaturated fats, at least as long as the latter two are consumed in moderation. Both polyunsaturated and monosaturated fats come with a variety of benefits for you. Polyunsaturated fats, which are otherwise known as your essential fatty acids, improve your blood cholesterol levels, along with your triglyceride levels. They tend to be very good for your heart health (Leal, 2021). Take omega-3 fatty acids, which are a kind of polyunsaturated fat. Omega-3 fatty acids are excellent for improving your heart health and strength.

Omega-3 fatty acids can primarily be found in fatty fish like salmon, walnuts, flaxseeds, and canola oil. You can meet your body's omega-3 needs by eating fish two to three times a week if your diet permits it. Polyunsaturated fats, in general, can be found in fish, walnuts, flaxseed, canola oil, soybean, corn, and sunflower.

As for monounsaturated fats, they're known to be extremely beneficial for your heart. In fact, they can be credited for making scientists and the general public realize that fats weren't all bad. Until the 1960s, the general consensus all around was that fat was bad. Then, in the 1960s, some scientists noticed that individuals living in the Mediterranean region and, therefore, eating a Mediterranean diet had very low rates of heart disease compared to the rest of the world. This was puzzling to them because the Mediterranean diet, as you might know, is heavy on olive oil. So how come all that olive oil wasn't damaging people's hearts?

The answer to that question became obvious after a little bit of study: Olive oil wasn't bad for you because it contained monounsaturated fats, and monounsaturated fats looked out for your heart rather than hurt it. Of course, olive oil isn't the only ingredient in the world that contains monounsaturated fats. Other food products do as well. Chief among these are peanut oil, canola oil, avocados, nuts of any kind, and seeds.

Incorporating Nutrient-Dense Fats Into Your Diet

You'd think that more people would be aware of the importance of eating essential, healthy fats, yet that's not necessarily the case. In fact, most people don't eat enough healthy fats. For instance, experts agree that about 8-10% of your caloric intake should come from polyunsaturated fats (Harvard School of Public Health, 2018).

So, how can you make sure to incorporate more healthy, nutrient-dense fats into your diet? The first thing you need to keep in mind is that fats are obviously high in calories. They're so high in calories, in fact, that you get about 9 calories from a gram of fat, whereas you only get 4 calories from a gram of protein or even carbs (Bhirani, 2023). So, as helpful and healthy as they are, they need to be consumed in moderation. As a rule, your daily fat consumption should equal about 20-35% of your daily caloric intake, as you might remember.

Your fat sources, meanwhile, need to be healthy ones. Avocados, fatty fish such as mackerel, salmon, and sardines, nuts, and seeds are great options to go with. This isn't just because of the health benefits that the fats in these foods have to offer you. It's also because good fats actually promote muscle growth by improving your cholesterol levels. You see, the process of repairing microtears and building new muscle fibers begins with healthy fats. When you eat healthy fats, you increase your good cholesterol levels. When your good cholesterol levels increase, they trigger a mechanism in your body that releases your growth hormones. Your growth hormones flood through your system and get to work growing your muscles. In the process, they trigger amino acids, which are vital for crafting muscle fibers (*How to Choose Good Fats for Building Muscle*, 2021).

When choosing your fat sources for muscle building, you need to go for the most nutrient-dense ones, meaning ones that are high in other substances like proteins. Your first go-to in this regard is eggs, if your diet permits it, or tofu. Eggs have a lot of calories to offer you, and they're very nutrient dense. Their protein levels are quite high, for one. They have plenty of leucine—an amino acid—for instance, which is an especially good building block for new muscle fibers. Eggs' vitamin B levels are pretty high as well, which is good news since vitamin B helps your body generate more energy during workouts. The one caveat with eggs is that they have some degree of saturated fats in them, too. Hence, it's important to not overdo it with them, at least if you don't want your bad cholesterol levels to start climbing.

Salmon is another top fatty resource choice for you, at least if you're a pescatarian. Rich in omega-3 fatty acids, salmon is obviously rich in protein. The same can be said of tuna. The only difference with tuna is that its mercury content can be rather high. So, it must be consumed with some moderation, too.

Next up, you have avocados. The grand majority of the calories you can get from avocados come from fats. However, avocados aren't all that high in calories, which means you can eat them without having to worry too much. An avocado does have some protein to offer you—4 grams of it, to be specific—but it's packed with vitamins K, C, B, and E.

Another valuable resource for you to take advantage of is nuts and seeds. The good news with nuts and seeds is that you have a very broad range of options to choose from, and you can mix and match to your heart's content. Walnuts, chia seeds, and flaxseeds should be on your priority list, though, since they contain especially high levels of omega-3. You should remember, though, that nuts are very high in calories, so it would be best to not overdo it with them.

Embracing Hormonal Balance and Recovery

As you've already seen, healthy fats are absolutely necessary for anyone looking to build muscles since they facilitate the release of the hormones that are necessary for muscular growth. However, that is not the only hormonal process in which essential fats take part (Lang, 2017). Actually, healthy fats play a part in the production of so many different hormones that it wouldn't be a stretch to say they're necessary for the ability to maintain your hormonal balance. Take insulin, for instance. Insulin is a hormone that your body produces to process sugar—that is to say, carbs—and turn it into fuel. At the same time, it helps keep your blood sugar levels from suddenly spiking and crashing. If your body can't produce enough insulin, then you might eventually develop type 2 diabetes, which you obviously want to avoid.

What does insulin have to do with healthy fats, then? Well, specific types of fats increase insulin sensitivity, making it easier for you to maintain healthy blood sugar levels. The type of fat that's capable of doing this are your good friends, omega-3 fatty acids. Omega-3 fatty acids can increase your insulin resistance by reducing inflammation across your body. That is one of the many benefits that they have to offer you. They can also keep your stress levels from rising by blocking the production of the stress hormone known as cortisol. This can ward you against conditions like chronic anxiety, which can develop when you have an excess of stress hormones in your system.

Going back to insulin for a moment, insulin sensitivity isn't just important for the sake of your blood sugar levels. It's important for you to be able to avoid developing some types of cancer, too. When your blood sugar levels end up being too high, you end up with excessive body fat. This often leads to rapid cell growth and throws your hormone system out of balance. When this happens, the odds of there being abnormal cell divisions throughout your body suddenly increase (Strommen, 2020). In other words, your risk of developing some kind of cancer increases. At the same time, your immune system stops being able to work as well because, like your hormone system, it needs healthy fats to perform at optimal levels. Having a weakened immune system means not being able to kill off any germs that enter your body, much less eliminate those cancerous cells that suddenly start forming after all.

Healthy fats also play a pivotal role in the production of two hormones known as progesterone and estrogen. This is because unlike all our other hormones, which are made of proteins, our sex hormones—meaning estrogen and testosterone—are made out of fats. So, when your fat intake proves too low to produce these hormones sufficiently, your sex drive starts going down, as do your serotonin levels. In search of a quick fix, you start craving carbs since they will trigger a quick but short-term release of this hormone. This will undeniably make you start feeling better, but the effects will wear off all too quickly. Pretty soon, you'll be craving carbs again, which will result in your exceeding your daily suggested carb intake levels, all while you're still suffering from a fat deficiency.

Chapter 8:

Strategic Supplementation for Vegans

What if your plant-based diet of choice is veganism, meaning you're foregoing certain foods like fatty fish and eggs? Are you likely to experience any nutritional gaps in this case? While eating a vegan diet won't usually mean you will experience some kind of nutritional deficiency, as long as you eat as varied a diet as possible, there is a small possibility that you might. This is especially true in cases where you're being more restrictive with your diet. So, as a vegan, there are eight specific deficiencies you might experience down the line. These are

- protein and amino acids
- omega-3 fatty acids
- vitamin B12
- vitamin D
- iron
- calcium
- zinc
- iodine (Ryan, 2021)

Knowing what your nutritional needs are when it comes to these eight items can help you to plan accordingly and keep you from experiencing any deficiencies. Knowing what the signs of a deficiency are, on the other hand, can help you to remedy the situation before it becomes too damaging for you.

Identifying Potential Nutritional Gaps

The first and most glaring nutritional gap you might be experiencing is one of proteins and, thus, amino acids. It might be that you're not eating as much protein as you should. Maybe you are eating plenty of protein but aren't getting all nine essential amino acids that you need. You might think you are eating all the protein you need to be eating since you're eating the same amount as a meat eater (Hobson, 2021). Eating the same amounts of different foods—plant-based proteins and animal meat—doesn't mean getting the same amount of protein, though. Different kinds of foods have different nutritional content, as you've witnessed for yourself. This is the primary reason why you should always check the nutritional content of the foods you're going to eat. It's also why you need to consume a wide variety of plant-based proteins.

You can tell that you're experiencing a protein deficiency if (*Are You Getting Enough Protein?*, 2022) if

- your hair and nails have gotten brittle
- you get sick often,
- you often feel hungry and weak,
- you're having difficulty thinking, or you experience mood swings,
- you're experiencing muscular weakness, or
- stress fractures start happening in your bones.

Should you notice one or more of these signs, the first thing you'll need to do is evaluate your daily protein intake carefully. Then, you can focus on protein combinations that would provide you with all nine amino acids that you need. You might also consider getting some plant-based protein powder and making protein shakes, which make for great mid- and postworkout snacks, if you'll recall.

As a vegan, you might also experience an omega-3 fatty acid deficiency. This is because omega-3 fatty acids exist in the highest quantity in fatty fish like mackerel. You might be experiencing a deficiency if you're not eating enough walnuts, seeds, and the like to get all the omega-3 your body needs. Signs that you're experiencing a deficiency will be

- skin and hair problems like dry skin and brittle hair,
- difficulty sleeping and feeling fatigued,
- experiencing joint pains and muscle cramps,
- having difficulty focusing and maintaining your attention,
- having memory troubles that are out of the ordinary,
- experiencing an uptick in your allergy symptoms,
- heart problems, or
- prolonged and heavy periods with lots of clotting (*Omega-3 Deficiency Symptoms & How to Get Enough*, 2019).

Vitamin B12 is most often found in animal meat. There aren't a lot of plant-based foods that have an abundance of B12, which is a shame because this vitamin is vital for DNA synthesis and thus is used for cell reproduction. Without it, things can go pretty wrong with these processes. You can tell that you have a deficiency if you

- feel extremely tired and lethargic,
- keep experiencing pins and needles,

- have developed ulcers in your mouth,
- are experiencing muscular weakness,
- are having trouble with your vision,
- are experiencing depression or general confusion, or
- are having memory problems.

As for how you can correct the deficiency, you can do so by taking vitamin B12 supplements. Alternatively, you can add fortified foods like soy products and milk alternatives to your diet, as they will be rich in these vitamins.

A second vitamin deficiency you might experience on a vegan diet is vitamin D. True, your skin can generate vitamin D through sun exposure, but there are limits to that, especially if you spend most of your day indoors. Normally, you'd replenish your vitamin D stores by eating things like fatty fish, egg yolks, and milk. Deprived of these options, you might start feeling the lack, the symptoms of which are

- an inability to fall asleep or sleep well,
- general fatigue and muscular weakness,
- aching bones or bone pain,
- hair loss,
- having pale skin,
- losing your appetite, or
- depression or general feelings of sadness (*9 Vitamin D Deficiency Symptoms*, n.d.).

Should you notice the signs of this deficiency, you can immediately get to work remedying it. That will mean eating more of certain plant-based foods that have high vitamin D content, such as nondairy milk—

that is to say, milk substitutes—and mushrooms, which are high in vitamin D3. In addition to that, you can take vegan supplements. Most vitamin D supplements are made from sheep's wool. So, if you're looking for a vegan alternative, you'll need to go with algae-derived vitamin D3 supplements (Ryan, 2021).

As a vegan, you might also experience certain mineral deficiencies. An iron deficiency is a common enough example. Iron is absolutely vital for your red blood cells. Iron is found in hemoglobin, which is tasked with carrying oxygen throughout your body. Without iron, it cannot perform its job as well. This is the main reason why people suffering from an iron deficiency become anemic. They can also experience symptoms like fatigue and depression. Truthfully, iron can be found in various plant-based products, like spinach. However, the iron levels of plant-based foods are typically lower than that of animal meat. Hence, you might experience a deficiency even if you eat foods that contain iron. A sound way to fix this matter is to eat more iron-rich foods such as legumes, nuts, seeds, and leafy greens. An even better way is to eat such foods with ingredients that have a high vitamin C content since vitamin C makes it easier for your body to absorb iron.

Yet another mineral deficiency you might experience is one of calcium, especially since you'll be cutting things like milk and cheese out of your diet. You can tell you're experiencing a calcium deficiency if you are experiencing things like

- memory loss,

- general confusion,

- tingling hands, feet, or face,

- muscle spasms and cramps,

- brittle or weak nails,

- depression,

- hallucinations, or

- brittle bones that fracture easily (Kahn, 2019).

Once you've been given a calcium deficiency diagnosis, you'll be able to fix it by upping your intake of fortified milk substitutes since they will be high in calcium. Fortified oat milk, soy milk, almond milk, and rice milk should be your go-to options here. You can similarly add more nuts, seeds, and leafy greens to your diet and start taking calcium supplements.

Likewise, you might experience a zinc deficiency as a vegan, which will have troubling implications for your immune system. Zinc plays a key role in keeping your immune system strong and healthy and helps your body to synthesize proteins. There are a number of plant-based foods that are rich in zinc. The problem is a fair bit of those, like legumes, bread, and cereal, contain something called phytates. Phytates tend to bind zinc, making it hard for your body to absorb it. Given that, you need to consume double the amount of zinc-filled foods that a nonvegan or nonvegetarian would consume in order to achieve optimal zinc levels.

You can tell you have a zinc deficiency if you're experiencing

- hair loss,

- brittle nails.

- eye problems and eye infections.

- slow-to-heal wounds.

- loss of sense of taste.

- loss of sense of smell. or

- diarrhea (*Zinc Deficiency*, 2022).

You can fix your zinc deficiency by taking supplements and eating more zinc-rich foods. You can also break down phytates before you eat your zinc-rich foods. To do this, you'll have to soak foods like beans in water for an hour or two before cooking them. The water should break the phytates in your legumes down, thereby increasing your access to zinc.

The last deficiency you might experience as a vegan is one of iodine. An iodine deficiency would immediately affect your thyroid, causing it to swell. This is a condition known as goiter, whose own characteristic symptoms are difficulty swallowing, trouble breathing, and even a choking sensation. Other non-goiter-related symptoms might be

- puffy skin,
- a hoarse voice,
- dry and scaly skin,
- general confusion,
- infertility, or
- thinning, coarse hair (Nicole, 2022).

As a vegan, you might experience an iodine deficiency as a result of cutting seafood and dairy out of your life. If you have such a deficiency, then the best and easiest way to remedy it is to add iodine salt to your diet. You can also start using seaweed or kelp as an ingredient in your dishes, as it will be high in iodine. Seaweed must be consumed in moderation, though, as its iodine levels may, in fact, be too high. Of course, you can also take supplements or make sure to eat bread that has been made with either calcium iodate or potassium iodate or pasta that has been cooked in water with iodized salt in it. You can eat more of certain fruits, too, that are high in iodine, such as bananas, cranberries, prunes, strawberries, and cranberries. Add to that some high-iodine vegetables, namely zucchini, watercress, potatoes, green beans, spring greens, corn, and kale, and things should be right as rain.

Vegan-Friendly Supplements for Muscle Building and Fat Loss

Since there are a variety of deficiencies you might experience as a vegan, there are a variety of supplements you might consider taking regularly. One of the chief deficiencies you might experience is B12, as you'll recall. Experts recommend that all adults, including you, take 2.4 mcg of vitamin B12 per day. This is what's known as your recommended daily allowance (RDA). If you're going to be taking B12 supplements to meet your RDA, then you're going to have to get a kind of over-the-counter pill that you'll place under your tongue. Said tablet will then melt. Alternatively, you can get a prescription nasal spray. Most people prefer lozenges, though; nasal sprays aren't necessarily the most pleasant thing in the world (Boyers, 2021).

Next, you might add a daily iron supplement to your list. If you're an adult man between the ages of 19 and 50, you're going to want 16 mg of iron per day. If you're an adult woman in the same age range, you're going to want to take 36 mg of iron since women typically require more iron. If you're 51 years old or older, however, you'll need 16 mg of iron a day, regardless of your gender. Having said all that, you should always watch the iron content of the foods you're eating carefully, especially if you're taking a supplement. It is vital that your iron levels do not exceed 45 mg a day, lest you start experiencing some serious health complications.

Then there's vitamin D. Vitamin D is another daily supplement you might consider as a vegan, especially if you're used to staying indoors for most of the day. If you're between the ages 16 and 71, then your RDA of vitamin D is 600 IU, regardless of your gender. If you're 71 years old or older, on the other hand, your RDA is 800 IU. There are a number of different vitamin D supplements out there, but the best one for you will be either a D3 or a cholecalciferol supplement. This is because these two supplements are the easiest ones for your body to absorb out of all the options that are available to you. Of these, D3 will be the better option because it won't be made from sheep wool and thus will be vegan.

Vitamin D3 is often combined with vitamin K. Combining the two is a practice that some people follow when taking vitamin D supplements, especially if they are vegan. This is because vitamin D and vitamin K work together synergistically to support various aspects of your health. Vitamin D is crucial for calcium absorption and bone health, while vitamin K plays a role in directing calcium to the bones and teeth and away from arteries and soft tissues. This helps prevent the buildup of calcium in blood vessels, which can contribute to arterial calcification. Meanwhile, vitamin D helps the body absorb calcium, making it available for bone mineralization. Vitamin K2 activates proteins that help bind calcium to the bone matrix. Together, they promote better bone density and reduce the risk of osteoporosis and fractures. By preventing calcium from accumulating in blood vessels, vitamin K2 may have a protective effect on cardiovascular health, too. Vitamin D also plays a role in maintaining healthy blood pressure and reducing inflammation.

Next up is omega-3. Your RDA for omega-3 will change depending on whether you're a man or a woman. If you're an adult woman, you're going to need 1.1 grams of omega-3 per day, whereas if you're a man, your RDA is going to be 1.6 grams. While your daily intake could surpass these limits a little bit, you shouldn't consume more than 4 grams of omega-3 since doing so can raise your cholesterol levels. As a vegan, the type of omega-3 supplement you'll want to go with will need to be made from algae, as opposed to fish, so be sure to check the labels of what you're getting so that you know that's the case.

Having cut milk and dairy products out of your life, you might experience a calcium deficiency, too, and seek to remedy it with supplements. How much calcium do you really need, though? Well, a man between the ages of 19 and 70 will need 1,000 mg of calcium. A woman between the ages of 19 and 50 will need that same amount of calcium. Meanwhile, women over the age of 51 will need 1,200 mg of calcium, while men over the age of 71 will need to consume 1,200 mg of calcium.

As for what type of calcium supplement you'll need to take, calcium supplements come in a variety of forms, the least expensive of which is calcium carbonate. This type of supplement will need to be taken with the food you eat. Otherwise, your body won't be able to absorb calcium properly, even if you take your supplements every single day.

As for zinc, your RDA for this will be 8 mg for adult women and 11 mg for adult men. You should typically try to not exceed these measures. You should especially avoid going over 40 mg of zinc per day since that could lead to some serious health issues for you.

Finally, you might consider taking an iodine supplement of some sort and liposomal vitamin C. Your RDA of iodine will be 150 mg per day, whether you're a man or woman. Like zinc, consuming too much iodine can be quite harmful for you. Hence, your daily intake should not exceed 1,100 mg per day at most.

Maximizing Absorption and Effectiveness

It's great that you know which supplements you can take and how much of certain substances you need in your system. But is there anything you can do to increase how well your body is able to absorb vitamins or how effective those supplements will be? Actually, there are. For starters, supplements should always be taken with meals that preferably include some kind of essential fat, like the ones found in avocados or olive oil. Fats play an important part in the absorption process of vitamins, as you'll recall. So, taking vitamin supplements with fats will hasten the process of their absorption (Munoz, 2022).

Other kinds of supplements, meanwhile, like iron, for example, should be taken with water. This is because such supplements are water soluble as opposed to fat soluble. In other words, it's water that helps them to be better absorbed by your body, not fats.

Just as there are certain substances you should consume with supplements, there are ones that you should avoid eating or, more accurately, drinking with them. Chief among those substances is alcohol. You should never take alcohol with your supplements as it will affect their effectiveness and solubility. You also should never take supplements with coffee. As a rule, there should be at least an hour-long window between when you take your supplement and have that first sip of coffee. This is because coffee contains caffeine, and caffeine is the kind of stimulant that can affect supplement absorption very easily.

Last but not least, you should also avoid smoking while you're taking your supplements. The chemicals that you inhale when you smoke, you see, can affect how well your body is able to absorb supplements, too. In fact, you should quit smoking altogether, if you're able to since it comes with many health hazards. The damage that smoking causes to your lungs and respiratory system cannot be understated. Given that, it can be argued that smoking is a practice that can hinder your efforts to work out since it reduces your lung health and capacity. As a result, it'll reduce the effectiveness of your workout sessions, too, making it harder for you to build muscle, lose fat, and meet whatever fitness goals you've set for yourself.

Chapter 9:

Effective Training Strategies

By now, you already know that you need to set fitness goals for yourself and develop some kind of fitness plan to be able to meet those goals. The kind of plan that you devise will determine whether you're successful in your efforts to build muscle and get into shape the way you want to. The reason for this is quite simple: Different kinds of training strategies lead to different kinds of results. If you want to bulk up, for instance and are mostly doing cardio exercises, then the odds are that you are not going to be able to meet your workout goals. You'll be able to lose weight, but building muscle the way you aim to will be a challenge because you're not working out your muscles the way you need to for optimal muscle growth. For this, you will need to do strength training exercises regularly. Not only that, but you'll need to adopt the right kind of training exercises and strategies that will meet your body's specific needs and lead you to the endpoint you want to reach bit by bit.

Designing Resistance Training Programs for Muscle Gain

There's one specific type of exercise that's good for building muscle, and that's strength training. Otherwise known as resistance training, strength training is a workout method where you provide your muscles with some kind of resistance to go up against to get them to contract repeatedly. In doing so, you cause microtears to form over your muscles, which then get healed through the natural processes of your body, where new muscle fibers are built to fix those tears. Those muscle fibers build on top of one another, creating new layers of muscles, resulting in you bulking up.

Strength training can involve either the use of your body weight or actual weights. This type of training needs to provide you with some challenges if it is to be effective. Otherwise, the training won't cause the microtears you need to be formed, and nothing much will change throughout your body. Luckily, there are several things you can do to make sure your workout provides you with the challenge you need, like

- gradually increasing the heaviness of the weights that you work out with as your muscles grow and get used to your old sets of weights;

- gradually increasing the number of sets and reps you do in lieu of increasing the weights you're working with, thereby ensuring you're still challenged by them;

- gradually increasing the difficulty of the exercises you're doing or graduating to harder exercises, like moving from modified push-ups and planks to actual push-ups and planks;

- increasing your training frequency; or

- reducing your rest time between your sets (*Resistance Training – Health Benefits*, 2012).

As you're designing your fitness plans and the strategies that you will be adopting for them, you're going to have to bear certain rules in mind, that is, if you really do want to build muscle. The first of these rules is that you need to create a workout regimen that is made up of different types of exercises that work different groups of muscles. This way, you'll be able to ensure uniform muscle growth and won't skip leg day, to borrow an old joke.

Another rule to consider is to use different types of resistance as you're working out. Working out with weights is a great way of training your muscles, but so are using springs, your own body weight, and items like resistance bands. These will work your muscles in different ways and help them get stronger in different manners.

Your next rule is to always try to introduce new exercises or moves to your training routine. This can keep your training program from becoming boring or monotonous. Getting bored while you're working out can be disastrous because it can eat away at your motivation and sense of discipline. Boredom can lead you to make up excuses about why you can't work out that day. That skipped day can quickly turn into two, then three... Before you know it, it will have been weeks since you last worked out. Keep introducing new exercises, workouts, and activities to your training program, though, and you'll be able to keep things fresh. You'll provide yourself with new challenges to rise to, and efforts to do so will stave off any boredom you might have otherwise felt.

Rule number four is to take regular breaks between your sets. You might be disinclined to do this since "rest" sounds like it's akin to "laziness." However, nothing could be further from the truth. Resting between sets is crucial for working out because not only does it give your muscles the momentary break they need to recuperate, but it also gives you the time you need to get your pulse and breathing rate under control, hydrate, and even eat a snack to replenish your energy.

Now that you know what your key workout rules are, the question is, "What training strategies do you need to go with?" Your first strategy is to work "big." That means opting for movements and exercises that work multiple muscle groups and joints at once, as opposed to just a single one, the way bicep curls do. That's not to say you can't do bicep curls or smaller movements like that—you can and you should—but your strategic priority should be bigger movements.

Bigger movements are colloquially known as multijoint movements. Multijoint movements are great because they allow you to lift greater weights, which gives you a greater challenge. The bigger the challenge, the greater the muscle growth, as long as it's a realistic challenge for your current fitness level, of course. To that end, movements like squats, bench presses, planks, and deadlifts are great multijoint exercises to go with.

Going off of the "greater the challenge, greater the gain" rule, another strategy to adopt is to train heavy. Training heavy—while taking the appropriate safety measures, like having someone spot you, for example—is a good idea because it makes your muscles contract eccentrically and concentrically. This stimulates your muscles more, causing greater microtears across your muscles, which ultimately equals greater build. One way to ensure you're training heavy is to go for a minimum of 10 reps per set and go up to 15, if you can. For multijoint movements, you can go for fewer reps—between three and 10, to be specific—since you're putting strain on practically your whole body for those. One example of a training routine that follows this rule might be (Campbell, 2010)

- three to five reps of your first exercise, done in four sets or

- 10-12 reps of every movement you execute thereafter, done in three sets, with the last set going to fixing any failure of form.

Training heavy is important. In fact, you should always go hard. The logic behind this strategy is fairly simple: You want to work out every day, but you don't want your workouts to lead to fatigue and exhaustion. The only way you can ensure that doesn't happen is if you train different muscle groups on different days. Training hard every day is a good idea, as long as you work different muscle groups, giving the ones you don't work a chance to heal the microtears they've already incurred.

A good measure of whether or not you're going hard enough—or not hard enough, for that matter—is how you feel after a training session. If you're feeling tired but good, then you're doing it right. If, on the other hand, you're dead and feel pretty unable to move, then you're probably overdoing it and should reduce the intensity you're working out at for a bit. This goes especially for individuals who are new to working out. If you haven't ever worked out or if you haven't done so in a while, then gunning it right off the bat will be a bad idea. Your body, unused to the intensity you're going for, will quit after just a short while. Alternatively, you yourself will, on a mental level, start making up excuses as to why you can't work out. This is why it's important you gauge your fitness level and start out slow, progressively increasing the difficulty of your exercises as you gain more strength and endurance without injuring yourself.

Once you have your routine selected and practice correct form, you may want to adopt the strategy of utilizing progressive overload in your workouts. Progressive overload is about improving the way in which you execute the moves of an exercise. With progressive overload, you have to option to stick with the exact same weights you had started off with but change up other factors while focusing on perfecting your moves. For instance, you can shorten the rest time you have between sets. Alternatively, you can increase the number of sets you do, you can increase weights, or you can increase training frequency and intensity as you keep going. You can even increase the number of sets you do. Hence, you can start out with three sets the first round, then increase that to five, and then to six, if you want to. In doing so, you'll progressively overload your muscles—hence the name—and give them a proper challenge.

Of course, increasing your reps and sets will not mean much if you're moving through your movements too quickly. Resistance training moves cause your muscles to tense up. As a rule, you want to hold that tension for a little bit. This is why you want to execute your moves slowly and in a rhythm. It's also why you want to keep that rhythm consistent, no matter how much you may want to pick up speed. To avoid this, you must always push yourself to do your exercises slowly and strive to keep going at that same speed at all times. That way, you'll be able to keep your muscles under tension for longer and maximize the effects of your training.

Incorporating Cardiovascular Training for Weight Loss

Resistance training is obviously great for building muscle. However, it's not necessarily ideal for weight loss, even if it can help with it. There is one type of exercise that's great for weight loss, though, and that's cardiovascular training. Cardiovascular training, or cardio, as it's largely called, is the given name for exercises that get your blood pumping really fast (Waehner, 2019). When you're doing cardio, you typically sweat heavily and breathe quite quickly. Your heart starts beating really fast, too, and all of those things get you to burn through a lot of calories. Understandably, the higher your heart rate gets, the more calories you burn.

Having said that, some cardio exercises are better for weight loss than others. One cardio exercise to try is high-intensity interval training (HIIT). As per the name, HIIT involves short periods of very high-intensity activity followed by periods of low-intensity activities (Team Acko, 2022). In this type of training, low-intensity periods are generally followed by short rest times to allow your body to recover before picking things up with high-intensity periods again.

Then there's low-intensity steady-state (LISS) cardio, which creates caloric burn as long as you do it correctly and consistently. This is because slow steady cardio preserves muscle tissue but burns fat. LISS cardio burns glycogen as its first energy source until it realizes that the demand on your muscles is not too great, and it turns to its secondary source of energy—your fat reserves. Recommended cardio includes activities like power walking, using machines like the Stairmaster, the flat or uphill treadmill, the elliptical, and jogging, running, or cycling. Aim for at least 30 minutes of such activities each day and add five more minutes each week until you reach 60 minutes. To burn fat, cardio should be performed at 70-80% of your maximum heart rate (MHR) MHR= 220-age multiplied by intensity %. For example, MHR= 220- 48 years old X 70%= 120 bpm.

Running is another great cardio exercise for you to go with. Going for a run is the type of exercise that's known for its ability to burn fat. It's also known for how it can get you to build muscle and, thus, gain strength. Overall, running can boost your heart health significantly and even improve your mood and mental health in the process. How many calories you burn while running will depend entirely on how long and far you run.

The one caveat with running is that it does put some impact on your knee joints. Hence, it can cause them to ache a little bit, especially if you've gone running without proper running shoes. If this is a problem that you're struggling with, then you can always try jogging rather than running. Alternatively, you can opt for walking instead. Walking is a very low-impact activity, which means that, unlike running, it puts little to no stress on your knees. Of course, walking doesn't mean going for a leisurely stroll since that wouldn't get your heart rate climbing in any way. Rather, it means keeping up a brisk pace. Walking regularly can be a great activity for you, seeing as it can reduce your risk of developing type 2 diabetes, improve your heart health, and lower your blood pressure, all while helping you lose weight.

Cycling can be another option to consider, one that you can do outdoors on a bike or indoors by going to a spin class or something of the sort. Like walking, it's a low-impact sport that can improve your heart health. Interestingly enough, it can also strengthen your bones and even make your abdominal muscles get toned since the movement cycling involves works those muscles too.

To cap your list of ideal cardio exercises, there's rope jumping. Rope jumping is a full-body exercise, which is just one reason why it can quickly help you shed fat. It's the type of activity that makes your heart rate climb, thereby enabling you to burn a lot of calories.

Chapter 10:

Recovering as a Plant-Based Athlete

The kinds of foods you eat and the supplements you take obviously play a vital role in your health, as well as your ability to lose weight and build muscle, as you've already seen. The kinds of exercises you do and how you go about doing them obviously play a major part in this, too. There's a third factor, however, whose role in these processes is just as important, and that's getting the rest you need. The importance of rest and recovery on your fitness journey can't be overlooked, not if you want to get into shape the way you want to. You might be hesitant to take a proper rest, thinking that resting means being lazy. That, however, isn't the case. Resting means giving your body the time it needs to recover and heal itself properly.

Remember those microtears that form while you're working out? Well, it takes time and energy for your body to get to work fixing them and knitting new muscles over them. Should your body be denied that time, it won't be able to heal your muscles. Those microtears, then, will still be in place when you head in for your next workout session. Far from being healed, they'll either get larger or new tears will be added on top of them. Keep this cycle going for long enough, and you'll be damaging your muscles at a much faster rate than your body can heal them. Hence, instead of experiencing new muscle growth, you'll come face-to-face with muscle breakdown.

Again, you avoid all of this if you simply give your body the time it needs. What exactly does that mean, though? How much time does your body truly need to rest, and what does "rest" look like? Is there anything specific you should be doing during those rest periods to augment the healing processes that are going through your body? Are there any plant-based recovery techniques and strategies that you can use to hasten your recovery?

Prioritizing Sleep and Health

The short answer to all those questions is "yes." The real answer, though, is lengthier than that because there are several things you need to do to ensure you get the proper amount of rest to support your body's healing and recovery. One of the most important things you need to do is to get regular sleep. Sleep might sound like it's completely unrelated to muscle building, but it's actually an important part of the process. You see, your body needs to release certain growth hormones for new muscle fibers to be created and for new muscles to be built. Those growth hormones are released throughout your body while you're sleeping. Hence, they repair the microtears across your muscles during that time period as well.

Your body won't be able to do any of this if you're not getting enough sleep, though. What do we mean by "enough" sleep? That depends on your specific needs and the kind of lifestyle you lead. However, a regular adult who is not trying to build muscle will usually need between seven and nine hours of sleep per night (Tan, 2023). An adult who is trying to build muscle, on the other hand, will need close to a good nine hours of sleep.

It should be mentioned that there is a stark difference between a restful nine hours of sleep and a fitful one. The quality of your sleep plays just as important a part in muscle growth as quantity, you see. When you get restful sleep, when you enter into deep sleep mode, your muscles produce more growth hormones. When you sleep fitfully, on the other hand, they are unable to do this because the hormone production and release processes that take place while you sleep get interrupted. So, you end up with fewer of those hormones, which ends up meaning your recovery takes longer than it should.

Taking measures to develop good sleeping habits, then, is a great idea. One way you can do this is to cut back on things like caffeine and other similar stimulants. Refraining from drinking coffee and other caffeinated drinks after a certain time of the day will help with this. Ceasing any and all strenuous activity at least two hours before you go to bed can help improve the quality of your sleep, too.

Another strategy you might adopt to give your body all the recovery time it needs is to take naps. Napping might seem like a lazy thing to do, but like sleeping, it is something that kickstarts the production of growth hormones in your body. On top of that, napping actually slows down your body's metabolic rate, thereby increasing the blood flow to your muscles. This means that when you nap, more growth hormones and oxygen are delivered to your muscle cells, which further promotes both muscle growth and muscle health.

That being said, napping can never take the place of a full, decent night's sleep, and more to the point, it shouldn't. The ideal strategy to adopt where naps are concerned would be to take short power naps throughout the day and then get nine hours of sleep per night. This way, you can maximize the effects of the muscle growth process. You can also take advantage of one of the additional benefits that naps have to offer, which is that they can reduce both inflammation in your muscles and lower your stress levels.

Managing Stress and Cortisol Levels

Speaking of stress, lowering your stress levels is very important for your muscle-building purposes, too. This is because chronic stress can hinder your muscle-building efforts. Stress can stop you from building muscle because your body releases a hormone known as cortisol when you become stressed. Cortisol is a kind of hormone that blocks various bodily functions. This is because it's released as part of your fight-or-flight instinct. Your fight-or-flight instinct kicks into gear when you sense a threat. Back in our caveman days, that threat would usually be something lethal, like a sabertooth tiger in the vicinity. The cortisol starts flooding through your body when you see the tiger. Your heart starts beating faster, your muscles tense, and the blood flow to your extremities—your arms and legs—suddenly increases. These allow you to do one of two things in that situation: fight the tiger or run away from it.

The problem with the fight-or-flight instinct these days is that we no longer live near sabertooth tigers. In fact, we hardly live near any predators at all. Yet, we still get stressed for a variety of reasons. It's perfectly fine for you to feel stressed from time to time—everyone does—but stress becomes a problem when it becomes chronic. If you have chronic stress, that means you're constantly stressed, which also means that cortisol is flowing through your body. Hence, cortisol is constantly shutting down and blocking various bodily functions. Cortisol does this so that you won't waste energy unnecessarily and instead be able to use all that energy to fight or flee from the sabertooth tiger that's supposedly in the area. Since there are no tigers or predators in the area, though, cortisol effectively does this for no reason whatsoever. In other words, it blocks off your bodily functions, including your body's ability to generate new muscle, unnecessarily.

Not only does cortisol prevent muscle recovery and growth, it also causes muscles to break down. Since one of cortisol's functions is to get your body the energy it needs to flee or fight, it tries to do whatever it can to get you that energy as quickly as possible. Often, that results in cortisol actively breaking down muscle protein and having it converted into glucose so that it can be used as fuel. This process is known as muscle atrophy, as you may recall. Being chronically stressed, then, means experiencing muscular atrophy at a near-constant rate. That, in turn, means that you can't build muscle effectively.

Cortisol doesn't stop there. On top of causing your muscles to break down, it encourages your body to store more fat in your hips, belly, and thighs. Add to that how cortisol keeps you in a constant state of alertness, thereby making it difficult for you to fall asleep and stay asleep, and you can see why stress is the enemy of muscle building. You can also see why you need to take measures to deal with and lower your stress levels in a healthy way.

There are a myriad of ways you can go about achieving this. One of them is making sure to eat a healthy and balanced diet. Get all the micronutrients and macronutrients you need into your body—which you can do with a plant-based diet, as you've seen—and those nutrients will neutralize the harmful molecules that will be produced in your body while you're stressed (*Nutrition and Stress*, 2021). Furthermore, maintaining a healthy diet will keep your blood sugar levels balanced. That's good news since low or spiking blood sugar levels are known to worsen stress and increase your cortisol production.

Another way you can manage your stress is to avoid overtraining. When you overtrain, you often deny your body the recovery time it needs for both muscle growth and achieving optimal health (Gutknecht, 2022). Studies show that individuals who overtrain have higher levels of cortisol in their systems than individuals who don't. Given that, giving yourself rest days, where the only activity you do is go for a brisk walk, is an abundantly good idea.

If you're looking for other activities to do during your rest times, then trying relaxing activities such as yoga, deep breathing, and meditation is the way to go. Meditation is a simple, proven way of reducing stress and dismissing chronic anxiety from your life. It can reduce your rapid heart and breathing rates, reduce any negative emotions you may be feeling, lower your blood pressure, and improve the quality of your sleep. The same can be said for deep breathing exercises, which are part of meditation, and yoga, which is a meditative exercise in and of itself. These days, there are a number of apps, podcasts, and videos you can use to get into meditation.

The key to reaping the stress-relief benefits that meditation and other such activities have to offer is to do them consistently. If you're doing meditation, you should be doing it every single day. That way, you'll turn it into a habit, one that you can turn to whenever you feel your stress levels start rising. Having never meditated before, you might find it challenging to sit there for a full 20 minutes and focus solely on your breathing and the sensations you're feeling in that moment. That's perfectly normal. What you can do in this case is to start with a short meditation session that's perhaps five minutes long. After about a week or two, you can up your time to 10 minutes and then to 15 minutes (Mayo Clinic Staff, 2022). After more time goes by, you'll be able to meditate for 30 minutes in one sitting. That's not to say that your mind won't ever wander away and chase after intrusive thoughts. When it does, though, you'll be able to gently direct it back to the present moment without any judgment or harshness.

Plant-Based Recovery Techniques and Strategies

Let's go back to nutrition for a moment. You've already seen how beneficial a balanced plant-based diet can be for you and how it can help with muscle growth. You've also seen that it can further support muscle growth by lowering your cortisol levels. Is there anything else that balanced nutrition can do to support you during your recovery time? Put another way, are there any plant-based recovery techniques and strategies you can adopt to make this process easier?

By now, you likely won't be at all surprised to find out that there are plenty of plant-based recovery techniques for you to consider. The first and most obvious of these strategies is to pay close attention to postexercise nutrition. The snacks and meals you eat after you're done with your workouts clearly can make a huge difference in your endeavors to build muscle. Given that, eating snacks and meals that are very rich in protein, complex carbs, and electrolytes following your workout sessions is a fantastic idea. Making mixed GI—food with varying glycemic indexes—superfoods a part of that meal, and all your meals for that matter, is an even better one (*How to Maximise Post-Exercise Recovery*, n.d.).

The term GI is an acronym that stands for glycemic index. Foods can have low, medium, and high glycemic indexes. Now, when you work out, you burn through a lot of energy. You need to replenish all that energy by eating the right carbs. A sound way of doing this is eating a mix of low, medium, and high GI foods because these combos will be quicker to revitalize your glycogen reserves. Of course, you shouldn't just go with foods with different GI contents but ones that are nutritionally dense as well. To that end, you can combine various types of fruits and enjoy them together. You can pair bananas and dates, for instance, with foods that are very nutritionally dense, such as goji berries, blueberries, strawberries, and acai berries. In doing so, you can quickly reintroduce all the carbs and nutrients you need to your body and optimize your recovery process.

Another strategy to consider adopting may be taking probiotics (LaRue, 2017). Probiotics can be considered a kind of supplement that is fantastic for your gut health and digestion. They support the good bacteria that exist in your gut and help them to do their jobs better. They help fix any damage that might have been done to your gut bacteria by things like refined sugars and trans fats, which are notorious for killing off gut microbiota. By taking probiotics, you can support your digestive system and, in the process, increase its ability to synthesize the nutrients you're giving it, like proteins, which can then be used to support your body's efforts to rebuild your muscles. If you don't want to take probiotics in supplement form, you can always incorporate foods that have plenty of probiotics in them. Fermented foods such as kimchi, yogurt, miso, kefir, tempeh, sauerkraut, and kombucha will be perfect for this.

A final strategy to consider might be to eat more foods that have antioxidants—or phytochemicals as they're otherwise known. By eating foods that have strong antioxidant properties, you can reduce the inflammation that'll occur in your muscles after your workouts.

Chapter 11:

Troubleshooting and Overcoming Plateaus

Anyone who has ever worked out before knows that there are times when you can hit plateaus. Plateaus are times when you seemingly aren't making any kind of progress at all. You see this often with weight training, where, at first, you make a lot of progress but then hit a certain point where you don't seem to be able to get past a certain weight threshold. You keep pushing yourself and keep trying, but there's no apparent, visible change to be seen. Pretty soon, your routine ceases to be challenging for you, and you feel like there's nothing you can do about it.

A similar kind of plateau can happen with weight loss, where you'll still be sticking to your plant-based diet but won't be able to observe any more changes. This will prove frustrating, and if you let it get to you, it can cause you to quit the diet you're on. You might experience that same kind of frustration when you hit a weight-lifting plateau, too. Understand why these plateaus happen, though, and you can take some measures to address their root causes. In doing so, you can keep your frustration from building and deterring you from quitting your workout routine or diet. Instead, you can figure out solutions or workarounds to the problem at hand and keep going.

Identifying Common Challenges in a Vegan Diet

Vegans often hit weight loss plateaus because their metabolisms slow down after a certain point or because they have become a bit sloppy, for lack of a better word, and therefore aren't adhering to the rules of their diet as strictly as they used to (*Vegan Weight Loss Plateau?,* 2021). To start with the former, as a vegan, your metabolism might have slowed down as part of your body's survival mechanism. Human beings used to be hunter-gatherers, as you know, and as hunter-gatherers they never knew where their next meal was coming from, nor did they know how much they'd get to eat. Because of this, the human metabolism evolved to slow down and burn less fuel upon noticing that it was getting less food, which you typically do when you're on a diet.

The second reason you might have hit a weight loss plateau is that you're not adhering to your diet in the same way that you used to. There's a difference, after all, between breaking the rules every once in a while and becoming lax with how you play things. If you're giving yourself a "treat" that you really shouldn't every single day, then that's going to impact your weight loss and muscle gain efforts.

There are several strategies you can adopt to overcome weight loss plateaus. The first of these is to cut a few hundred more calories from your diet. I suggest cutting 100 calories at a time, reassessing your progress after a week, and cutting an additional 100 until you reach your goal. Take care not to dip too low in calories, or you could risk your health, injure yourself, or feel run down. That way, you can potentially restart the weight loss process by forcing your body to dip into your fat reserves and use them as energy sources. At this stage, this won't be all that hard for you. You likely won't even miss the calories you're cutting out of your diet. A 100- or 200-calorie deficit from your typical daily intake should be enough to get things going again.

Increasing your daily activity level a bit more could be another strategy to consider. Extending your workout sessions by 10 or 15 minutes, for example, could work wonders by getting you to shed more calories. Going on daily walks can work wonders, too, especially if cardio isn't part of your workout routine yet.

One rather unexpected strategy might be to take a two-week break from the diet you're on. That doesn't mean starting to eat meat all of a sudden, but it does mean letting go of the general rules and restrictions for a period. That's a good idea because it gets your body to relax for a bit and restarts your metabolism in the process. Once your two weeks are up, you can get back into your diet and realize that you're now able to lose weight without any issues once more.

Adjusting Nutrition and Training for Continued Progress

As for weight-lifting plateaus, these typically occur because your body has gotten used to and adjusted to your exercise routine. That's actually a good thing because it's plain evidence of how much progress you've made. Seeing further progress, though, will require making further adjustments to your training schedule and being persistent.

One adjustment might be to increase the intensity of your workouts a bit. This is because making your muscles work harder is absolutely necessary for overcoming plateaus. That can mean doing higher numbers of sets or increasing the weights you work with while maintaining the correct form at all times, of course.

Another adjustment you might try is to vary your exercise routine. Studies show that varying your routine can increase your ability to gain new muscles by about 11.6-12.2%. Meanwhile, keeping your workout routine constant results in lower rates of muscle gain, those rates being stuck around 9.3% specifically (Quinn, 2022).

While you're varying your routine, you might consider cutting exercises that you've outgrown from your schedule. If you've been doing modified push-ups and see that they've now gotten too easy for you, then cutting them out of your program and replacing them with something harder is a good idea. So is cutting toe raises, which are good for initially building up your calves since you can only make so much headway with them.

One reason you might have hit a plateau is that you're not giving your body the time it needs to rest and, thus, release the growth hormones that are necessary to facilitate muscle growth. Giving your body more time to rest and prioritizing sleep should help with this. This measure should also recharge your mental and emotional reserves, thereby keeping you motivated and energized to keep going.

Mental Strategies to Stay Motivated

Speaking of motivation, keeping yours up is essential if you are going to stick to your workout and dietary routines permanently. Otherwise, you'll either eventually get bored and quit, or you'll get frustrated the moment you hit a plateau and quit rather than trying to push through.

Luckily, there are a couple of secrets to keeping your motivation levels up, and all of them are pretty simple. One is to set fitness goals for yourself (Hernandez, 2022). Setting fitness goals gives you a concrete target to strive for, which can increase your dedication and determination by leaps and bounds. As long as you set realistic, SMART goals for yourself, of course. At the same time, meeting goal after goal can be very satisfying while helping you keep track of your progress.

Sometimes, you need a little outside help for motivation, be it in the form of competition or encouragement. That being the case, finding a gym buddy to work out with might be a good idea. Having a gym buddy can make your workout sessions social and fun. Furthermore, a gym buddy can be a source of encouragement, keeping you from skipping a workout day because you don't feel like it.

A workout mentor can do a similar thing, of course. Unlike a gym buddy, though, such a mentor won't provide you with competition. They will, however, provide you with something to strive toward. Having a mentor can be inspiring, both because you'll have an example to look up to and because you'll have someone to talk to and get advice from whenever you're struggling with something.

This might seem like a simple solution, but preparing the perfect workout playlist can be rather motivating, too. Music is known for its ability to put you into a certain mindset and mood. Hence, creating a playlist filled with music that can get you pumped up and eager to keep going, such as *Eye of the Tiger*, can be a fantastic strategy to adopt.

Your final motivational strategy is a rather obvious one: Pick workouts, activities, and exercises that you actually enjoy doing. If you hate going to the gym but insist on working out there, odds are, your fitness journey won't last long. If, on the other hand, you love swimming, then making this activity a part of your weekly routine will only prove uplifting for you. You will, therefore, be a lot more likely to stick with it and, thus, infinitely more likely to achieve whatever fitness goals you've set for yourself.

Conclusion

As you have seen again and again throughout *Plant-Based Body Transformation*, building muscle, shedding fat, losing weight, and getting into shape while maintaining a plant-based diet isn't out of the realm of possibility. In fact, these are easier goals to achieve than what most people believe, that is as long as you follow a few basic rules. These rules, as you've again no doubt seen, are quite simple and reasonable when you think about it. You have to keep your protein intake high so your body can build new muscle. You have to keep your carb intake high to ensure you have all the energy you need to both work out and build muscle. You similarly have to consume an adequate amount of fat so that your body can absorb all the nutrients you need and keep your body functioning as it should.

Likewise, you have to eat a varied diet to make sure you're getting all the different kinds of nutrients your body needs. While you're doing that, you have to work out regularly to build muscle and lose weight. You have to make sure your workouts provide you with some kind of challenge. Otherwise, you won't be able to develop your muscles in the way that you want.

Aside from all that, though, there's one final thing you need to do, and that's to celebrate all your achievements as you walk down this plant-based path, even the smallest ones. As you work out, your strength, conditioning, and flexibility are all going to improve over time. As they do, you're going to meet milestone after milestone. The thing is, some of these milestones are going to be pretty small and, therefore, easy to miss, at least if you aren't paying attention to them. They will, however, build on top of one another, leading you to even bigger milestones and culminating in you achieving your fitness goals.

Achieving your fitness goals will take some time. So, if you aren't seeing and recognizing the milestones you meet along the way, you might start feeling like you're not making any progress at all. This obviously won't be true, but it will feel true enough to you. That feeling will, unfortunately, be quite disheartening. So much so that it can easily cause you to give up on your fitness goals and quit trying.

This, right here, is why you need to celebrate any and all milestones you achieve. By celebrating even the smallest milestones you meet, you'll make your progress immediately visible to yourself. Thus, you'll get to encourage, energize, and motivate yourself significantly.

Since you'll be keeping your motivation levels up, you'll both be able to stick to your workout routine more and enjoy it a lot more, too. In the process, you'll get to see the very transformation that you're undergoing. You'll get to become a firsthand witness to how your body changes and evolves bit by bit, day by day, until one day you find yourself looking in the mirror, smiling, and asking, "Is this really me?" This transformative process, however, starts with but a single step. The question you have to ask yourself is whether you're ready to take that initial step. Think carefully, then: Are you ready to go after and embrace the change that you have been seeking and transform not just your body but your life in the process?

Bonus Chapter:

Recipes

Having discussed the various plant-based ingredients and foods you can enjoy along your fitness journey, we'd be remiss not to share a couple of choice recipes for you to try. While you can come up with a variety of new recipes using a bit of creativity, here are our favorite ones:

Recipe: Vegan Chili

Prep Time: 7 minutes

Cook Time: 20 minutes

Total Time: 27 minutes

Nutrition Facts:

Calories: 83

Protein: 4 grams

Carbs: 18 grams

Fat: 1 gram

Ingredients:

- 1 cup of rinsed green lentils
- 1 cup of rinsed garbanzo beans
- 1 cup of rinsed kidney beans

- 1 chopped white onion
- 4 minced garlic cloves
- 1 tsp. of cumin
- 1 tsp. of chili flakes
- 1 tsp. of coriander
- 1 1/2 tsp. of salt
- 1 tsp. of pepper
- 2 tsp. of chopped cilantro
- 1 diced green pepper
- 1 tbsp. of Worchestershire sauce
- 1 block of firm tofu

Instructions:

1. Take an instant pot and turn it on to the sauté setting to heat up 1 tbsp. of olive oil in it.
2. Chop up your onion as the oil warms and toss it in to sauté for 3-5 minutes.
3. Add in the minced garlic and stir, cooking for an additional 30 seconds.
4. Add in all the remaining ingredients, except for the tofu, mix them well, and close the pot's lid. Let the ingredients cook together for 10 minutes.
5. Run the mixture through the blender to achieve a thicker consistency if you want to. If not, leave it as is.

6. Release the pressure of the instant pot, then remove the lid and stir in the tofu.

7. Serve yourself a bowl of chili, chop up your cilantro, and use it as garnish before enjoying your dish.

Recipe: Overnight Oats

Prep Time: 5 minutes

Cook Time: 3+ hours

Total Time: 3+ hours and 5 minutes

Nutrition Facts:

Calories: 370

Protein: 13 grams

Carbs: 59 grams

Fat: 17 grams

Ingredients:

- 1/2 cup of rolled oats
- 1/2 cup of oat milk
- 1 tbsp. of maple syrup
- 1 tsp. of ground cinnamon
- 1 tsp. of chia seeds
- 1 cup of blueberries (or fruit of your choice)

Instructions:

1. Fill a mason jar with oats and pour the oat milk inside.

2. Mix in all your other ingredients and close the jar's lid.

3. Place the jar in the fridge and let it sit for at least three hours, ideally overnight.

4. Take out the jar in the morning and enjoy.

Recipe: Scrambled Tofu

Prep Time: 5 minutes

Cook Time: 10 minutes

Total Time: 15 minutes

Nutrition Facts:

Calories: 774

Protein: 18.2 grams

Carbs: 11.4 grams

Fat: 7.7 grams

Ingredients:

- 1 block of firm tofu
- 2 tbsp. of salsa
- 1 tbsp. of turmeric
- 1 crushed garlic clove
- 1/2 tsp. of onion powder
- 1 tbsp. of nutritional yeast
- 1/4 cup of mushrooms

- 1/4 cup of diced spinach leaves
- 1/4 cup of diced peppers of your choice

Instructions:

1. Heat up 1 tbsp. of water in a skillet over medium heat and sauté all your vegetables for 5 minutes.
2. Dice up your tofu and drain the pieces on a paper towel for 3 minutes.
3. Crumble the tofu and toss the crumbles in the skillet to cook them.
4. Add in the onion powder, nutritional yeast, and salsa, and keep cooking for another 3 minutes.
5. Cook everything together for an additional minute and serve.

Recipe: 6 Ingredient Lentil Salad

Prep Time: 15 minutes

Cook Time: 5 minutes

Total Time: 20 minutes

Nutrition Facts:

Calories: 255

Protein: 12 grams

Carbs: 31 grams

Fat: 10 grams

Ingredients:

- 2 cups of rinsed green lentils

- 1/2 cup of halved cherry tomatoes
- 1 cup of shredded white cabbage
- 1/3 cup of sliced cucumbers
- 1/3 cup of halved and pitted calamata olives
- 1/4 cup of diced kale
- 1/2 tbsp. of Dijon mustard
- 1/2 cup of extra virgin olive oil
- 1/4 cup of lime juice
- Salt and pepper to taste

Instructions:

- Chop up all your vegetables and mix them together in a bowl.
- Add in your rinsed lentils and mix well.
- In a smaller bowl, mix together your Dijon mustard, olive oil, lime juice, salt, and pepper.
- Pour the mixture over your larger bowl with the other ingredients in it and mix well.
- Serve and enjoy.

Recipe: Bean Burger Patties

Prep Time: 10 minutes

Cook Time: 15 minutes

Total Time: 25 minutes

Nutrition Facts:

Calories: 90

Protein: 5 grams

Carbs: 16 grams

Fat: 1.5 grams

Ingredients:

- 2 cups of rinsed black beans
- 1/4 cup of diced red onions
- 3 minced garlic cloves
- 1/3 cup of rolled oats
- 2 tbsp. of extra-virgin olive oil
- 1/4 tsp. of coriander
- 1/4 tsp. of Italian seasoning
- Salt and pepper to taste

Instructions:

1. Rinse your black beans and mash them down in a bowl, leaving 1/4 of the mixture semimashed, while the other portion is fully mashed.

2. Add in all your remaining ingredients and mix them together using your hands until they stick together.

3. If the mixture seems too wet, add more oats to firm it up and mix more.

4. Form your patties by hand.

5. Warm a skillet over medium heat and pour in 1 tbsp. of olive oil.

6. Once the olive oil has heated up, toss your patties in and cook each side for 3-4 minutes.

7. Let your patties cook for 5 minutes before serving.

Glossary

Adrenalin: A hormone that is secreted by your adrenal glands that speeds up your blood circulation, breathing rate, and metabolism, thereby preparing your muscles for hard work.

Amino acid: The building blocks that proteins are made up of and which are used by your body to repair muscular tears and build new muscle fibers.

Carbohydrates: An organic compound that your body uses as its primary energy source and that's obtained by eating starchy and sugary foods such as fruits and vegetables.

Cortisol: A hormone that's released in your body when your stress response kicks in that speeds up your heart and breathing rates and causes various functions in your body to shut down in order to direct more energy to the actions you'll be taking as part of your fight-or-flight instinct.

Enzymes: A substance that your body produces to kickstart various hormonal processes.

Estrogen: A sex hormone that is necessary for a woman's ability to maintain their reproductive and sexual health.

Fatty acid: The building blocks that fats are made of and broken down into once they're eaten that help the human body perform various functions like absorbing vitamins.

Glucose: A simple sugar that carbs are converted into and that's used as a fuel source in your body.

Metabolism: The biochemical process by which your body transforms the food you eat into energy for you to use or store.

Mineral: A kind of inorganic substance that your body needs to be able to perform at optimal levels.

Testosterone: A sex hormone that is necessary for a man's ability to maintain their reproductive and sexual health.

Vitamin: Kinds of organic substances that your body needs in various quantities in order to perform at optimal levels.

References

Adidas Runtastic Team. (2022, August 23). *Relieve sore muscles: 7 foods that help*. Adidas Runtastic Blog. https://www.runtastic.com/blog/en/sore-muscle-recovery/

Aoyama, S., Kim, H.-K., Hirooka, R., Tanaka, M., Shimoda, T., Chijiki, H., Kojima, S., Sasaki, K., Takahashi, K., Makino, S., Takizawa, M., Takahashi, M., Tahara, Y., Shimba, S., Shinohara, K., & Shibata, S. (2021). Distribution of dietary protein intake in daily meals influences skeletal muscle hypertrophy via the muscle clock. *Cell Reports*, *36*(1), 109336. https://doi.org/10.1016/j.celrep.2021.109336

Are you getting enough protein? Here's what happens if you don't. (2022, November 14). UNCLA Health. https://www.uclahealth.org/news/are-you-getting-enough-protein-heres-what-happens-if-you-dont

Bhirani, R. (2023, September 2). *Fats: Importance in nutrition and healthy ways to add fat to your diet*. Healthshots. https://www.healthshots.com/healthy-eating/nutrition/fats-in-diet/

Boyers, L. (2021, May 5). *The most important vegan vitamins and supplements*. GoodRx; GoodRx. https://www.goodrx.com/well-being/supplements-herbs/vegan-vitamins-and-supplements

Burke, N., Shannon-Hagen, M., & Karsies, D. (2015, April 9). *Plant-based diets: Why all the hype?* Rogel Cancer Center | University of Michigan. https://www.rogelcancercenter.org/living-with-cancer/mind-body-side-effects/nutrition/plant-based-diets-why-all-hype#:~:text=In%20terms%20of%20cancer%20prevention

Campbell, A. (2010, April 15). *10 tips for building muscle now*. Men's Health. https://www.menshealth.com/fitness/a19534499/10-muscle-building-tips/

Can you build muscle with plant-based protein? (n.d.). ProSupps.com. Retrieved September 5, 2023, from https://www.prosupps.com/blogs/articles/can-you-build-muscle-with-plant-based-protein#:~:text=Start%20Building%20Muscle%20with%20Plant

Carbohydrates - The master fuel. (2019, May 3). United States Department of Anti-Doping. https://www.usada.org/athletes/substances/nutrition/carbohydrates-the-master-fuel/#:~:text=Consuming%20carbohydrates%20during%20workouts%20lasting

Cheeke, R. (2021, May 12). *How to build muscle on a plant-based diet: Staple foods, meal plans, and philosophy*. No Meat Athlete. https://www.nomeatathlete.com/build-muscle-plant-based/#:~:text=In%20order%20to%20gain%20muscle

Chuang, S.-Y., Chiu, T. H. T., Lee, C.-Y., Liu, T.-T., Tsao, C. K., Hsiung, C. A., & Chiu, Y.-F. (2016). Vegetarian diet reduces the risk of hypertension independent of abdominal obesity and inflammation: a prospective study. *Journal of Hypertension, 34*(11), 2164–2171. https://doi.org/10.1097/HJH.0000000000001068

Clinton, C. M., O'Brien, S., Law, J., Renier, C. M., & Wendt, M. R. (2015). Whole-Foods, Plant-Based Diet Alleviates the Symptoms of Osteoarthritis. *Arthritis, 2015*, 1–9. https://doi.org/10.1155/2015/708152

Cook, B. (2021, December 3). *10 ways to track fitness progress*. Stamina Products. https://staminaproducts.com/blog/10-ways-to-track-fitness-progress/

de Groot, J. (2020, June 10). *Vegan diet muscle gain: The 10 best plant based protein sources | Tanita.eu*. TANITA EUROPE B.V.; TANITA

EUROPE B.V. https://tanita.eu/blog/10-plant-based-protein-sources-for-muscle-gain

English, N. (2020, April 11). *Best macros calculator for tracking muscle gain and fat loss*. BarBend. https://barbend.com/best-macros-calculator/

Espinosa-Salas, S., & Gonzalez-Arias, M. (2023). *Nutrition, Macronutrient Intake*. PubMed; StatPearls Publishing. https://www.ncbi.nlm.nih.gov/books/NBK594226/

5 steps to start a fitness program. (2019). Mayo Clinic. https://www.mayoclinic.org/healthy-lifestyle/fitness/in-depth/fitness/art-20048269

Greger, M. (2023, February 16). *The first studies on vegetarian vs. meat-eating athletes*. NutritionFacts.org. https://nutritionfacts.org/blog/the-first-studies-on-vegetarian-vs-meat-eating-athletes/

Gubbi, S., Hamet, P., Tremblay, J., Koch, C. A., & Hannah-Shmouni, F. (2019). Artificial Intelligence and Machine Learning in Endocrinology and Metabolism: The Dawn of a New Era. *Frontiers in Endocrinology*, 10. https://doi.org/10.3389/fendo.2019.00185

Gutknecht, L. (2022, February 4). *The effects of stress on muscle growth and how to reduce It*. Foodspring Magazine. https://www.foodspring.co.uk/magazine/effects-of-stress-on-muscle-growth#:~:text=Because%20recovery%20and%20muscle%20development

Harvard School of Public Health. (2018). *Types of fat*. The Nutrition Source - Harvard School of Public Health. https://www.hsph.harvard.edu/nutritionsource/what-should-you-eat/fats-and-cholesterol/types-of-fat/

Head, A. (2021, April 6). *8 pre-workout meals for the most energy and better results*. Women's Health.

https://www.womenshealthmag.com/uk/food/healthy-eating/g32138025/what-food-to-eat-before-a-workout/

Hernandez, M. (2022, December 20). *How to stay motivated to workout in 10 ways*. Chuze Fitness. https://chuzefitness.com/blog/ways-to-stay-motivated-to-workout/

Hobson, R. (2021, May 7). *Vegan diet: potential nutrition gaps and how to fill them*. Www.lifespanonline.co.uk. https://www.lifespanonline.co.uk/nutrition/vegetarian-and-vegan/vegan-diet-potential-nutrition-gaps/

How to choose good fats for building muscle. (2021, June 25). ISSA. https://www.issaonline.com/blog/post/how-to-choose-good-fats-for-building-muscle

How to eat complete proteins in vegetarian and vegan diets. (2022, August 22). INTEGRIS Health. https://integrisok.com/resources/on-your-health/2022/august/how-to-eat-complete-proteins-in-vegetarian-and-vegan-diets

How to maximise post-exercise recovery on a vegan diet. (n.d.). Naturya. Retrieved September 12, 2023, from https://naturya.com/blogs/superfood-news-and-education/maximize-muscle-recovery-on-a-vegan-diet#:~:text=A%20fantastic%20way%20to%20support

Jiang, X., Huang, J., Song, D., Deng, R., Wei, J., & Zhang, Z. (2017). Increased Consumption of Fruit and Vegetables Is Related to a Reduced Risk of Cognitive Impairment and Dementia: Meta-Analysis. *Frontiers in Aging Neuroscience*, *9*(18). https://doi.org/10.3389/fnagi.2017.00018

Kahn, A. (2019, July 31). *Hypocalcemia: Causes, symptoms, and treatment*. Healthline. https://www.healthline.com/health/calcium-deficiency-disease

Kim, H., Caulfield, L. E., Garcia-Larsen, V., Steffen, L. M., Coresh, J., & Rebholz, C. M. (2019). Plant-Based Diets Are Associated With a Lower Risk of Incident Cardiovascular Disease,

Cardiovascular Disease Mortality, and All-Cause Mortality in a General Population of Middle-Aged Adults. *Journal of the American Heart Association, 8*(16). https://doi.org/10.1161/jaha.119.012865

Lang, A. (2017, May 15). *10 natural ways to balance your hormones: Diet tips and more.* Healthline. https://www.healthline.com/nutrition/balance-hormones#healthy-fats

LaRue, K. (2017, August 18). *Tips to recover faster from exercise on a vegan diet.* BODi. https://www.beachbodyondemand.com/blog/recover-faster-on-a-vegan-diet

Leal, D. (2021, June 30). *How eating fat keeps you fit and healthy.* Verywell Fit. https://www.verywellfit.com/why-eating-fat-keeps-you-healthy-3121407

Mawer, R. (2017, June 12). *What is carb cycling and how does it work?* Healthline. https://www.healthline.com/nutrition/carb-cycling-101#the-science

Mayo Clinic Staff. (2022, April 29). *A beginner's guide to meditation.* Mayo Clinic. https://www.mayoclinic.org/tests-procedures/meditation/in-depth/meditation/art-20045858#:~:text=Meditation%20can%20give%20you%20a

Meyer, A. (2023, January 17). *How many carbs you should eat to build muscle.* EatingWell. https://www.eatingwell.com/article/8024634/carbs-to-build-muscle/#:~:text=Consume%208%20to%2010%20grams

Munoz, K. (2022, February 16). *Try these tricks to make your supplements more effective.* The Checkup. https://www.singlecare.com/blog/vitamin-absorption/#:~:text=Take%20fat%2Dsoluble%20vitamins%20at

National Heart, Lung, and Blood Institute . (2019). *Calculate your BMI - standard BMI calculator.* National Heart, Lung, and Blood Institute ; U.S. Department of Health & Human Services. https://www.nhlbi.nih.gov/health/educational/lose_wt/BMI/bmicalc.htm

National Research Council (US) Subcommittee on the Tenth Edition of the Recommended Dietary Allowances. (1989). Protein and Amino Acids. In *www.ncbi.nlm.nih.gov.* National Academies Press (US). https://www.ncbi.nlm.nih.gov/books/NBK234922/#:~:text=Nine%20amino%20acids%E2%80%94histidine%2C%20isoleucine

Nicole. (2022, September 15). *Vegan iodine sources and supplements: How to get enough.* Lettuce Veg Out. https://lettucevegout.com/nutrition/vegan-iodine/#:~:text=Vegan%20diets%20may%20be%20low

9 vitamin D deficiency symptoms (and 10 high vitamin D foods. (n.d.). University of Nebraska-Lincoln - University Health Center. https://health.unl.edu/9-vitamin-d-deficiency-symptoms-and-10-high-vitamin-d-foods

Nutrition and stress. (2021, September 23). University of North Carolina Chapel Hill - Campus Health. https://campushealth.unc.edu/health-topic/nutrition-and-stress/

NutritionED Contributor. (2022, November 30). *How to create a nutrition plan.* NutritionED. https://www.nutritioned.org/how-to-create-a-nutrition-plan/

Omega-3 deficiency symptoms & how to get enough. (2019, March 13). Camas Swale Medical Clinic. https://www.camasmedical.com/2019/03/13/omega-3-deficiency-symptoms/

Petre, A., & Ajmera, R. (2022, May 26). *The 18 best protein sources for vegans and vegetarians.* Healthline.

https://www.healthline.com/nutrition/protein-for-vegans-vegetarians#fruits-and-veg

Physical activity – setting yourself goals. (2012). Vic.gov.au. https://www.betterhealth.vic.gov.au/health/healthyliving/physical-activity-setting-yourself-goals

Plant-based diets. (n.d.). British Nutrition Foundation. https://www.nutrition.org.uk/putting-it-into-practice/plant-based-diets/plant-based-diets/#:~:text=A%20healthy%2C%20balanced%20plant%2Dbased

Quinn, E. (2022, May 19). *How to break through weight lifting plateaus.* Verywell Fit. https://www.verywellfit.com/six-tips-to-break-through-strength-training-plateaus-3120744

Raman, R. (2018, February 6). *When is the best time to take protein?* Healthline. https://www.healthline.com/nutrition/best-time-to-take-protein#TOC_TITLE_HDR_3

Resistance training – health benefits. (2012). Better Health Channel. https://www.betterhealth.vic.gov.au/health/healthyliving/resistance-training-health-benefits

Richards, J. (2023). *Albert Einstein said "Man was not born to be a carnivore."* Humane Decisions. https://www.humanedecisions.com/albert-einstein-said-man-was-not-born-to-be-a-carnivore/#:~:text=In%20a%20letter%20written%20to

Ryan, H. (2021, December). *9 nutrient deficiencies in began diets.* Life Extension. https://www.lifeextension.com/wellness/lifestyle/nutrients-deficiencies-vegan-diets

Satrazemis, E. (2022, December 7). *How much protein do I need to build muscle?* Www.trifectanutrition.com. https://www.trifectanutrition.com/blog/how-much-protein-do-i-need-to-build-muscle#:~:text=All%20of%20these%20recommendations%20fall

Sautter, D. (2023, March 21). *Does a plant-based diet for athletes help or hurt performance?* Adidas Runtastic Blog. https://www.runtastic.com/blog/en/plant-based-diet-for-athletes/

Sautter, D. J. (2023, July 5). *9 good carbs for muscle building (& when to eat them)*. Welltech. https://welltech.com/content/9-good-carbs-for-muscle-building-when-to-eat-them/

Strommen, L. (2020, January 16). *How dietary fat benefits hormones.* Women's International Pharmacy. https://www.womensinternational.com/blog/dietary-fat-benefits-hormones/

Talaei, M., Wang, Y.-L., Yuan, J.-M., Pan, A., & Koh, W.-P. (2017). Meat, Dietary Heme Iron, and Risk of Type 2 Diabetes Mellitus. *American Journal of Epidemiology, 186*(7), 824–833. https://doi.org/10.1093/aje/kwx156

Tan, C. (2023, April 14). *Do you need sleep for muscle growth?* Harley Street Medical Doctors. https://harleystreet-md.co.uk/blog/sleep-for-muscle-growth/#:~:text=Your%20body%20produces%20hormones%20crucial

Team Acko. (2022, November 28). *Best cardio exercises for weight loss.* Acko General Insurance. https://www.acko.com/health-insurance/health-guides/cardio-exercises-for-weight-loss/

10 mid-workout snacks to sustain performance. (2021, October 1). Health Fitness Revolution. https://www.healthfitnessrevolution.com/10-mid-workout-snacks-to-sustain-performance/

The plate method, a nutritionally balanced meal for vegans. (2022, January 28). Pick up Limes. https://www.pickuplimes.com/article/the-plate-method-26

Unlocking the power of macronutrient ratios: The key to your fitness goals. (2023, June 6). Sheru Classic World. https://sheruclassicworld.com/unlocking-the-power-of-macronutrient-ratios-the-key-to-your-fitness-goals/

Van Niekerk, T. (2023, March 27). *Meatless meals on the rise: Studying vegetarian statistics.* World Animal Foundation. https://worldanimalfoundation.org/advocate/vegetarian-statistics/

Vegan bodybuilding meal plan: Plant-based muscle gain. (2022, July 27). Steel Supplements. https://steelsupplements.com/blogs/steel-blog/vegan-bodybuilding-meal-plan-plant-based-muscle-gain

Vegan weight loss plateau? 3 reasons you're not losing weight. (2021, January 5). I Am Going Vegan. https://www.iamgoingvegan.com/vegan-weight-loss-plateau/#:~:text=Vegan%20weight%20loss%20plateaus%20often

Vitamin B12 or folate deficiency anaemia symptoms and treatments. (2019). National Health Service. https://www.nhsinform.scot/illnesses-and-conditions/nutritional/vitamin-b12-or-folate-deficiency-anaemia

Waehner, P. (2019). *Adding cardio to your workout routine to help with your weight loss.* Verywell Fit. https://www.verywellfit.com/cardio-for-weight-loss-1229851

What are macronutrients and micronutrients? (2022, October 5). Cleveland Clinic. https://health.clevelandclinic.org/macronutrients-vs-micronutrients/

Wirnitzer, K., Tanous, D., Motevalli, M., Wirnitzer, G., Leitzmann, C., Pichler, R., Rosemann, T., & Knechtle, B. (2022). Prevalence of Female and Male Vegan and Non-Vegan Endurance Runners and the Potential Associations of Diet Type and BMI with Performance—Results from the NURMI Study (Step 1). *Nutrients, 14*(18), 3803. https://doi.org/10.3390/nu14183803

Wood, C. (2020, June 28). *Carbohydrate recommendations for all activity levels.* Nutrigility. https://www.nutrigility.com/carbohydrate-recommendations-for-all-activity-levels/

Wu, H.-J., & Wu, E. (2012). The role of gut microbiota in immune homeostasis and autoimmunity. *Gut Microbes*, *3*(1), 4–14. https://doi.org/10.4161/gmic.19320

Yokoyama, Y., Nishimura, K., Barnard, N. D., Takegami, M., Watanabe, M., Sekikawa, A., Okamura, T., & Miyamoto, Y. (2014). Vegetarian Diets and Blood Pressure. *JAMA Internal Medicine*, *174*(4), 577. https://doi.org/10.1001/jamainternmed.2013.14547

Zinc deficiency. (2022, September 19). Health Direct Australia. https://www.healthdirect.gov.au/zinc-deficiency#symptoms

Made in the USA
Middletown, DE
09 November 2023

42135261R00071